Temporomandibular Joint Dysfunctio

Temporomandibular Joint Dysfunction
The essentials

R. G. Jagger BDS, MScD, FDS
Senior Lecturer and Consultant in Prosthetic Dentistry,
The Dental School, University of Wales College of Medicine,
Cardiff, UK

J. F. Bates BDS, MSc, DDS, DrOdont
Emeritus Professor of Restorative Dentistry
The Dental School, University of Wales College of Medicine,
Cardiff, UK

S. Kopp DDS, PhD
Professor of Clinical Oral Physiology,
Karolinska Institute, School of Dentistry, Huddinge,
Stockholm, Sweden

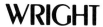

Wright
An imprint of Butterworth-Heinemann Ltd
Linacre House, Jordan Hill, Oxford OX2 8DP

℞ A member of the Reed Elsevier plc group

OXFORD   LONDON   BOSTON
MUNICH   NEW DELHI   SINGAPORE   SYDNEY
TOKYO   TORONTO   WELLINGTON

First published 1994

British Library Cataloguing in Publication Data

Jagger, R. G.
    Temporomandibular Joint Dysfunction:
    Essentials
    I. Title
    917.522

ISBN 0 7236 1015 0

Typeset by BC Typesetting, Warmley, Bristol BS15 5YD
Printed in Great Britain at the University Press, Cambridge

Contents

Preface

Whilst many textbooks have been produced on the subject of pain and dysfunction of the temporomandibular joint and masticatory musculature, most are of interest only to specialist workers. Undergraduates and practitioners have few readable textbooks which explain the aetiology, diagnosis and treatment of temporomandibular joint dysfunction in relatively simple terms. The present volume redresses the balance and provides an introduction to what is a complex subject that remains imperfectly understood, even by those who confine their professional lives to the treatment of patients suffering from temporomandibular disorders and chronic facial pain.

Acknowledgements

The authors wish to acknowledge the influence and guidance of Professor G E Carlsson who was the stimulus for the interest of RGJ and SK in the management of patients with joint dysfunction.

Thanks are due to the Dental Illustration & Audio Visual Aids Department, Cardiff Dental School, for their care and assistance in the preparation of the illustrations; to Mrs Gwen Allison for her patience in typing drafts and revisions and to Mrs Mary Seager of Butterworth-Heinemann for her support and encouragement.

Introduction

Temporomandibular disorders embrace a wide spectrum of specific and non-specific disorders that produce symptoms of pain and dysfunction of the muscles of mastication and temporomandibular joints. Examples of such specific conditions are rheumatoid arthritis, gout and condylar hyperplasia.

The term *temporomandibular joint dysfunction* is applied in a more restricted sense to the smaller cluster of related, relatively non-specific disorders of the temporomandibular joint and muscles of mastication that have many symptoms in common. The term temporomandibular joint (TMJ) dysfunction is used in this text as a synonym for TMJ dysfunction syndrome, TMJ pain dysfunction and facial arthromyalgia.

It must be emphasized that although non-musculoskeletal disorders in the orofacial region such as vascular, neoplastic or infectious diseases may produce similar symptoms, these are not considered to be temporomandibular disorders (McNeil, 1993). Thus symptoms of TMJ dysfunction are characteristically aggravated by chewing and other jaw movements but are independent of local disease involving the teeth, mouth or related structures.

It is generally accepted that the aetiology of TMJ dysfunction is multifactorial, in that several factors acting alone or in combination may be sufficient to cause the pathology of TMJ dysfunction. Both mechanical and emotional factors are regarded as being important. Specific factors include emotional stress, bruxism, trauma and dental malocclusion. Sometimes it is not possible to identify an aetiology positively.

Epidemiology

Epidemiological studies in many parts of the world confirm a very high prevalence of signs and symptoms of TMJ dysfunction. Most studies report at least 50% of individuals having at least one sign (e.g. masticatory muscle tenderness or joint clicking) although only 30% of subjects may be aware of such symptoms (Rugh and

Solberg, 1985). Symptoms of TMJ dysfunction are common in all age groups. Older age groups have slightly more symptoms than the young. Such studies may overstate the clinical significance of the problem because many symptoms may be mild and transient. Data from the USA however indicate that TMJ disorders may impose a significant health burden on the community. There are no great differences in frequency of symptoms of dysfunction between men and women in these epidemiologic populations. However, studies of patients attending clinics specializing in the treatment of TMJ dysfunction invariably record a female-to-male ratio of more than 2:1. Why this should be so is still a matter for conjecture. It is not believed that symptoms are more severe in women than men.

The peak incidence of symptoms in patients attending clinics for treatment is between the ages of 15 and 45.

The symptoms of TMJ dysfunction

Patients suffering from TMJ dysfunction complain of a variety of symptoms that may be present in various combinations which occur with varying severities and frequencies and which reflect the nature of the underlying pathology. Much remains to be learned about the symptoms of TMJ dysfunction, e.g. which symptoms have the most or least favourable prognosis. Signs and symptoms range from being mild, transient or self-limiting to severe and constant.

The commonly occurring symptoms are: pain, joint sounds, limitation of mandibular movements, ear symptoms and recurrent headache.

Pain

Pain may arise from TMJs and/or muscles of mastication. It is the symptom most commonly causing patients to seek treatment although joint sounds alone may be present. Pain may be present as a constant or periodic dull ache over the joint, the ear, the temporal fossa, at the angle of the mandible or around and behind the eye. Pain is usually elicited or aggravated by mandibular movement or by palpation of the affected region. The pain is often then reported to be sharp and more severe. Pain may also be more widespread, radiating to the neck and shoulder when the sternocleidomastoid and trapezius muslces are affected.

The aetiology of *myogenic pain* is poorly understood but it may be the result of two main factors—mechanical trauma and muscle fatigue (Klineberg, 1991). Both macrotrauma and microtrauma are described. Macrotrauma arises from an external force such as a blow to the face. Microtrauma arises in the absence of external force and is commonly associated with parafunction such as bruxism. Muscle fatigue is a complex physiological process that is also incompletely understood. Sustained static muscle contraction can cause localized ischaemia and an alteration in muscle fibre membrane permeability that results in local oedema. Specimens obtained from painful muscles by biopsy have demonstrated a non-serous inflammation due to mechanical microlesions of the interfibrillar connective tissue. The presence of a vascular inflammatory component can also be demonstrated sometimes by thermography. Localized tender areas of muscle which may be associated with firm bands or knots of muscles are known as trigger points. Pain arising from such affected muscles has been termed myofascial pain.

Articular pain can arise as a result of inflammation of articular and periarticular tissues caused by overloading or trauma to those tissues.

Inflammation of articular tissues as a result of degenerative changes such as occur in osteoarthrosis can also produce pain and sometimes it is impossible to distinguish early osteoarthritis from TMJ dysfunction.

Harris *et al.* (1993) postulated that mechanical or emotional stresses stimulate the release of neuropeptides. These can induce painful capsulitis, synovitis and myositis.

Joint sounds

Two forms of joint sounds are described:

(a) Crepitus (or crepitation). This is a grating or scraping noise that occurs on jaw movement which can be noticed by the patient and often can be palpated by the clinician. It is said by the patient to feel like sand-paper rubbing together. Crepitus is caused by the roughened, irregular articular surfaces of the osteoarthritic joint.

(b) Clicking. This is caused by uncoordinated movement of condylar head and the TMJ disc.

Several mechanisms have been suggested and it is probable that more than one is involved (Table 1.1).

Watt (1980) has proposed a useful classification of joint sounds which takes into account the nature of the sounds (click or crepitus), their quality (hard or soft), their position related to

Table 1.1 Causes of TMJ clicking (after Klineberg, 1991)

Dysfunction
(i)   Click associated with deviation in form of condyle, disc and temporal fossa
(ii)   Click associated with neuromuscular dysfunction
(iii) Eminence click
(iv)   Click (reciprocal) with anterior disc displacement
(v)   Click associated with hypermobility
(vi)   Tethered disc click

Cause
(i)   Remodelling and morphologic changes of the articular surfaces and disc perforations may provide mechanical obstruction to condylar translation
(ii)   Uncoordinated movement may be due to dysfunction of controlling muscles— the lateral pterygoid or masseter muscles. The mechanism of this is poorly understood
(iii) Eminence click occurs in association with a forced joint opening with a protrusive opening arc. This can occur unconsciously for example with a Class II occlusion or as a deliberate movement
(iv)   The antero-superior part of the mandibular condyle is normally related (in the closed mouth position) to the central fossa of the disc. The disc in some cases however may become displaced. Anterior displacement of the articular disc in the joint space causes a click to occur as the condylar head moves across the posterior ridge of the disc (Fig. 1.1b). This takes place on both opening and closing movements of the mouth. A double click is thus produced and is referred to as reciprocal clicking. (This condition may progress to 'closed lock' when the head of the condyle becomes unable to pass across the posterior ridge. This will result in limitation of opening of the mouth described below)
(v)   Hypermobility click occurs when the head of the condyle clicks over the anterior ridge of the disc when the mouth is very wide open
(vi)   Tethered disc click. A posterior disc attachment that has been damaged as a result of trauma may prevent the translation of the TMJ disc that should occur on opening of the mouth. Reciprocal clicking may occur as the head of the condyle passes over the anterior band of the meniscus on opening and closing of the mouth

mandibular movement (near, middle or wide) and whether the sounds occur on opening and/or closing of the jaws.

There is a need for more standardized clinical research, leading to classification of the various types of clicking and knowledge about changes in sounds with the course of time.

Limitation of mandibular movement

(a) MUSCULAR RESTRICTION

Muscular restriction is the most common reason for limitation of mandibular movement and is most often reflex in nature. The

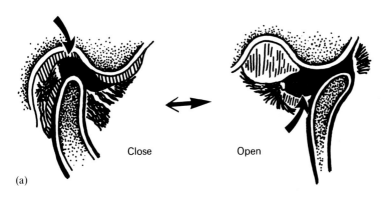

Close   Open

(a)

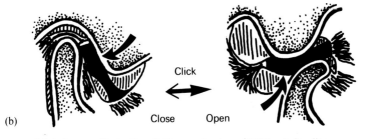

Click

Close   Open

(b)

Figure 1.1 A diagram illustrating clicking mechanism of TMJ anterior disc displacement. (a) Normal joint; (b) anterior disc displacement

restriction is caused by contraction in a group of muscles, and can be produced by forceful stretching of a muscle or its synergists (stretch reflex) or as a response to pain, either in the muscle or its synergists, or around the joint. Difficulties in opening the mouth after complicated tooth extractions and mandibular nerve blocks are difficult to explain, but might be caused by reflex muscular inhibition or intramuscular haemorrhage.

(b) DISC DISPLACEMENT—CLOSED LOCK

An anteriorly displaced disc may prevent the forward translation of the mandibular condyle. This results in limitation of opening of the mouth, i.e. closed lock (Fig. 1.2). Clinical signs are: reduced opening capacity, mandibular deviation on opening and tenderness to palpation of the affected temporomandibular joint. The early or

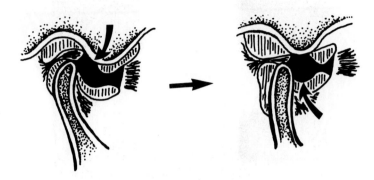

Figure 1.2 Anterior disc displacement without reduction (closed lock)

acute closed lock may result in interincisal opening of less than 35 mm. Progressive stretching of the posterior disc attachment may increase opening towards normal. Excessive stretching however may lead to thinning of the posterior of the disc and perforation of the posterior attachment (Fig. 1.3).

(c) LIGAMENTOUS RESTRICTION

The ligaments normally restrict the movements of the joint in all directions and operate when the muscles are unable to stop the movement and there is risk of dislocation of the joint, e.g. following sudden, violent movements. Sometimes ligaments become stretched and thus hypermobility results with possible sequelae, i.e. dislocation of the joint rather than restriction of movement. The sphenomandibular ligaments can sometimes be too short to permit a normal mouth opening capacity.

(d) DISLOCATION

On wide opening of the mouth the head of the condyle normally passes over the articular eminence. Occasionally a patient may be unable to close the mouth because the condyle cannot return into the fossa. The mouth is wide open and a feeling of panic is commonly described. The patient may eventually be able to reduce the dislocation himself or may present at hospital for treatment.

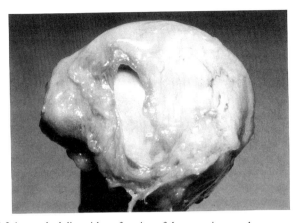

Figure 1.3 A stretched disc with perforation of the posterior attachment

Ear symptoms

Subjective ear symptoms are commonly associated with TMJ dysfunction (Koskinen *et al.*, 1980). Symptoms include tinnitus, itching in the ear, a blocked feeling and vertigo. The symptoms are probably due to functional disturbance of the Eustachian tube. It has been suggested that masseter hyperfunction can lead to vibration and clonus of the tensor tympani muscle which is also innervated by the trigeminal nerve. If internal ear disease is present in conjunction with TMJ dysfunction it is coincidental.

Recurrent headache

It is recognized that recurrent headache is a frequent accompaniment of pain and tenderness in the masticatory muscles. Headaches, however, should not be considered a symptom of TMJ dysfunction in the absence of other signs. Bruxism can produce temporal headache in the absence of other subjective symptoms but the temporal muscle is then usually tender to palpation and is often a symptom of generalized tension related to an associated anxiety state.

The association between recurrent headache, bruxism and symptoms of TMJ dysfunction is well recognized (Magnusson and Carlsson, 1978). TMJ dysfunction is most usually thought to be associated with tension type or (temporalis) muscle contraction headache, although an association with migraine headaches is also recognized (Steele *et al.*, 1991).

Chronic facial pain ('psychogenic' facial pain)

Symptoms of TMJ dysfunction are usually mild and self-limiting. If they become more severe, treatment may be required. Most symptoms are amenable to reassurance, advice or simple conservative treatment measures. Only occasionally should surgery be indicated for joint pathology.

A small group of patients with no joint pathology, experience chronic facial pain that is not well controlled by simple conservative treatment measures. Some of these patients are able to cope with the continuous unpleasant perception. If the coping mechanisms are insufficient, individuals may become depressed and focused on the impact of the pain, regardless of the original event that started the pain. They may then become complex chronic pain patients and require skilled, multidisciplinary management otherwise they are liable to go from one health care professional to another and become victims of multiple unsuccessful interventions (Tyrer, 1992).

Diagnosis and treatment of temporomandibular disorders

Dentists' knowledge of craniofacial anatomy and related disorders should enable them to diagnose temporomandibular disorders. The conservative management techniques including occlusal treatments described in this book should enable them to give advice and manage most patients. Only a few patients should need to be referred for specialist care.

Further reading

Ferrari M D and Lataste X (eds) (1989) *Migraine and Other Headaches.* Parthenon, Carnforth

Griffiths R H (1983) Report of the President's Conference on the examination, diagnosis and management of temporomandibular disorders. *Journal of the American Dental Association,* **106,** 75–77

Harris M, Feinmann C, Wise M and Treasure F (1993) Temporomandibular joint and orofacial pain: clinical and medicolegal management problems. *British Dental Journal,* **174,** 129–136

Klineberg I (1991) *Craniomandibular Disorders and Orofacial Pain.* Wright, Oxford

Koskinen J, Paavolainen M, Raivo M and Roschier J (1980) Otological manifestations in temporomandibular joint dysfunction. *Journal of Oral Rehabilitation,* **7,** 249–254

Magnusson T and Carlsson G E (1978) Comparison between two groups of patients in respect of headache and mandibular dysfunction. *Swedish Dental Journal,* **2,** 85–92

McNeill C (ed) (1993) Temporomandibular disorders. *Guidelines for Classification Assessment and Management. The American Academy of Orofacial Pain.* 2nd edn. Quintessence, Chicago

Moller E, Rasmussen O C and Bonde-Petersen F (1979) Mechanism of ischaemic pain in human muscles of mastication: intramuscular pressure, EMG, force and blood flow of the temporal and masseter muscles during biting. In: *Advances in Pain Research and Therapy, 3* (eds J J Bonica, J C Liebeskind and D G Albe-Fessard). Raven Press, New York, pp. 271–281

Rugh J D and Solberg W K (1985) Oral health disorders in the United States: temporomandibular disorders. *Journal of Dental Education,* **49,** 398–404

Steele J G, Lamey P L, Sharbey S W and Smith G M (1991) Occlusal abnormalities pericranial muscle and joint tenderness and tooth wear in a group of migraine patients. *Journal of Oral Rehabilitation,* **18,** 453–458

Tyrer S P (1992) *Psychology, Psychiatry and Chronic Pain.* Butterworth-Heinemann, Oxford

Travell J G and Simons D G (1983) *Myofascial Pain and Dysfunction: The Trigger Point Manual.* Williams and Wilkins, Baltimore

Wabeke K B, Hansson T L, Hoogstraten J and van der Kuy P (1989) Temporomandibular joint clicking: A literature overview. *Journal of Craniomandibular Disorders: Facial and Oral Pain,* **3,** 163–173

Watt D M (1980) Temporomandibular joint sounds. *Journal of Dentistry,* **2,** 119–127

2

The anatomy and function of the temporomandibular joint and muscles of mastication

The *stomatognathic system* is a term that has been used to describe the whole of the masticatory apparatus. Its use implies the need for an understanding of the inter-relationship between the various parts. This inter-relationship is important in that failure of integration between its components must lead to functional disturbances which in turn may cause pain in the muscles and joints and the associated problems of clicking, crepitus, etc.

There are standard text books that describe in detail the anatomy and physiology of the stomatognathic (masticatory) system.

Certain relevant applied aspects are revised in this chapter.

The temporomandibular joint

The joint comprises the inferior surface of the temporal bone, the mandibular condyle and the intervening disc. The articular surface of the temporal component comprises the glenoid fossa and that part of the articular eminence which extends from the sphenotympanic fissure to an area anterior to the most prominent part of the eminence (Fig. 2.1). Medially the joint extends to the suture between the articular part of the temporal bone and the greater wing of the sphenoid, with considerable individual variation in its dimensions and form.

The upper surface of the condyle presents a transverse ridge in the coronal plane, with a sloping surface extending anteriorly and posteriorly. These two surfaces converge to medial and lateral poles or bony prominences, to which are attached the capsule and the meniscus (Fig. 2.2).

The articular surfaces of both the upper and lower components of the TMJ are covered with fibrocartilaginous tissue which resembles that of the sternoclavicular joint. Both these joints possess a central disc or meniscus. The thickness of the fibrocartilage layer varies on the joint surfaces, being thickest on the articular surfaces which oppose one another, i.e. on the antero-superior of the condyle and

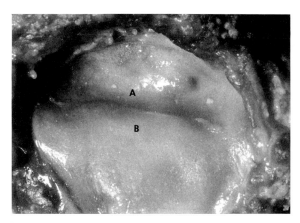

Figure 2.1 The temporal component of the TMJ: A articular eminence; B glenoid fossa

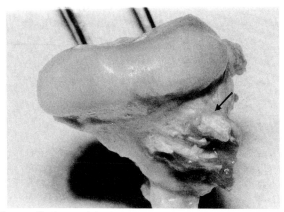

Figure 2.2 The mandibular condyle. Arrow points to attachment of lateral pterygoid to the neck of the condyle

on the infero-posterior surface of the articular eminence of the temporal bone.

The disc is made of a flexible, dense sheet of fibrous connective tissue, which is generally oval in shape. Its inferior surface is concave to fit the condyle, but superiorly the morphology is more complex. The posterior surface of the disc is convex to relate to the glenoid fossa, while anteriorly it is saddle-shaped, being slightly convex from side to side and concave antero-posteriorly to fit the eminence. From above it appears pear-shaped (Fig. 2.3) and has been described as resembling a schoolboy's cap, covering and extending forward in front of the condyle, to relate to the articular eminence of the temporal component. The varying thickness of the disc has led to the description of four distinct regions. These regions are: (1) the anterior band, (2) the intermediate zone, (3) the posterior band and (4) the bilaminar region. These zones are much wider in the transverse direction than in the antero-posterior direction on the upper and lower surfaces. The upper surface of the bilaminar zone is composed of two layers of fibro-elastic tissue. In subjects over 30 years, chondroid cells are often seen in the dense central part of the disc.

Attachments of the disc

Medially and laterally the disc is attached to the poles of the condyle, together with the enveloping capsule. Antero-medially the disc is attached to the anterior capsule ligament and also sometimes a few fibres of the lateral pterygoid. Posteriorly the bilaminar zone is attached to the posterior wall of the glenoid fossa and the squamo-tympanic suture and the lower layers to the posterior part of the mandibular condyle. A diagrammatic representation of a sagittal section of the joint is shown in Fig. 2.4.

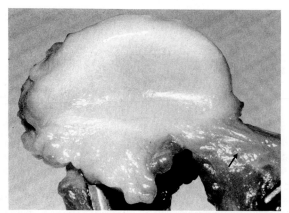

Figure 2.3 The TMJ disc. Arrow points to attachment of lateral pterygoid to anterior of disc

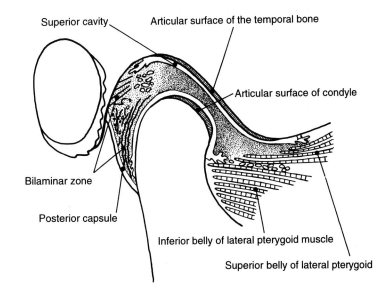

Figure 2.4 Diagrammatic representation of sagittal section through the TMJ

Function of the disc

Discs are present in many joints and have been considered to have the following functions:

- Shock absorption, protecting the articular surface.
- Increasing the congruity between the articular surfaces and thereby increasing the stability of the joint. The disc adapts itself to the varying curvatures of the different parts of the articular surfaces which engage in various planes of movement.
- Allowing a combination of different movements in the joint by dividing the joint into compartments and allowing the bony elements to move independently on the disc.
- Preventing undue forward gliding.
- A ball bearing action.
- Distribution of weight across the joint, by increasing the area of contact which may thus prevent wear.
- Assisting in lubrication of the joint.

The capsule and temporomandibular joint ligaments

The capsule is a thin, fibrous connective tissue sleeve that tapers from above down to the neck of the condyle. The capsule of the joint posteriorly and medially is ill-defined and posteriorly joins the fibrous tissue of the bilaminar zone. Anteriorly, the capsule is absent, and laterally the capsule is loose and thin, but is much stronger than on the medial aspect. The anterior part of the lateral wall is reinforced by the temporomandibular ligament, which is a dense collagenous band running posteriorly from the lateral surface of the zygomatic process of the temporal bone and the articular eminence on its route to the posterior and lateral surface of the neck of the mandible (Fig. 2.5). It is wider at its upper attachment on the zygomatic process and becomes triangular as it travels down to its insertion in the mandible. Movements of the mandible are also limited, to some extent, by the stylomandibular ligament and the spheno-mandibular ligament which are attached to the body of the mandible itself (Fig. 2.6).

The synovial membrane

The synovial membrane lining the periphery of the upper and lower joint compartments is folded, with villi-shaped structures which unfold as the joint moves (Fig. 2.7). When the condyle and disc move forward, the soft tissue of the posterior part of the disc is pulled forward. The amount of free synovial fluid lubricating the

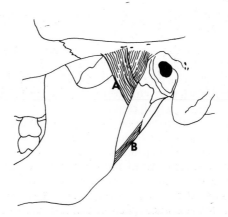

Figure 2.5 The joint capsule, lateral ligament (A) and stylomandibular ligament (B)

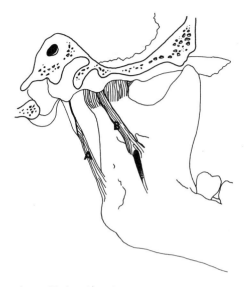

Figure 2.6 The stylomandibular (A) and the sphenomandibular ligament (B)

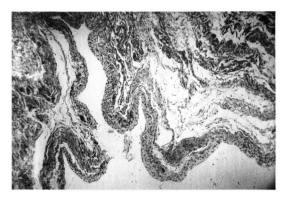

Figure 2.7 The synovial membrane

joint is scant and even when the joint is at rest and its potential volume greatest, no fluid can be aspirated from a healthy joint. Small amounts of fluid can be injected, 1.9 ml in the upper and 0.9 ml in the lower compartments to administer drugs, or contrast media for arthrography.

Synovial fluid

Synovial fluid is composed of a dialysate of blood plasma in combination with a mucopolysaccharide, namely hyaluronic acid. The synovial fluid has a very low protein content and some of this is bound to the hyaluronic acid, which is an asymmetric, long chain molecule of very high molecular weight. This polysaccharide is produced by a special type of synovial cell lining the synovial membrane.

The synovial fluid's main functions are lubrication, nutrition and clearance.

Blood supply to the joint

The blood supply to the TMJ comes from small branches of the superficial temporal and deep auricular arteries which supply the periosteum, muscles and tendons of the joint. The deep auricular artery supplies the anterior border of the capsule, and also the head of the condyle and via the nutritional foramina. A rich plexus of blood vessels surrounds the synovial membrane of the joint.

Innervation of the joint

The auriculo-temporal nerve supplies posterior and lateral branches to the capsule of the TMJ. There are further anterior articular nerves arising from the masseteric nerve as it enters the medial surface of the masseter muscle. From the proximal region of the masseteric nerve, where the deep temporal nerves take their origin, a few fine articular nerves arise which run down medially to innervate the anteromedial and medial aspects of the joint capsule and there are also branches of the lateral pterygoid nerve which also run through the muscle and innervate the antero-medial region of the joint capsule.

Mechanoreceptor nerve endings exist in the joint in a distribution which would be most effective for detecting changes in tension and are therefore most effective during masticatory and other joint movements. Some mechanoreceptors function as physiological receptors and are active during normal joint movements, whereas others activate only in extremes of joint movement and are normally totally inactive.

Adaptation of the TMJ to external forces

The articular tissue has a slow turnover of cells and intercellular material. During function, significant forces may be applied to the joint surfaces although only a small proportion of the forces generated by mastication are transmitted to the joints. The joint is capable of adaptation to these forces in three ways:

(i)   Alteration in the composition of the soft articular surfaces and metaplastic change of that tissue.
(ii) Restructuring of the osteons in the sub-articular compact bone and reorientation of the trabecular pattern.
(iii) Proliferation of articular tissues accompanied by changes in the external shape of the joint surfaces and the sub-articular bone.

There are limits, however, to the adaptive response. Exceeding these adaptive limits may lead to the degenerative changes of osteoarthrosis.

Muscles of mastication

The primary muscles of mastication are the temporalis, masseter and the medial and lateral pterygoids (Figs 2.8–2.10). These four muscles, together with the digastric, the mylohyoid and the genio-

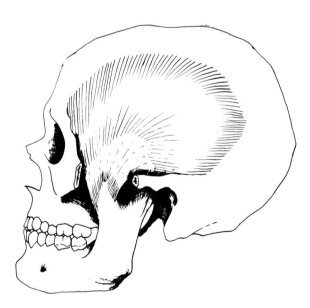

Figure 2.8 The temporalis muscle

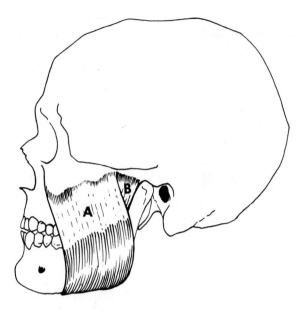

Figure 2.9 The masseter muscle: deep belly (A), superficial belly (B)

hyoid are responsible for movement of the mandible. The sterno-cleidomastoid and trapezius muscles may also be painful and tender to palpation in patients with symptoms of TMJ dysfunction.

It is important to be familiar with the applied anatomy of these muscles.

Innervation of the masticatory muscles

The trigeminal nerve is both the motor nerve for the muscles of mastication, and the sensory nerve for these muscles and the TMJ. The mandibular branch of the trigeminal nerve supplies branches to the masseter, the medial and lateral pterygoid and to the temporal muscles. A branch of the inferior dental nerve supplies the mylo-hyoid muscle and the digastric muscle.

Receptors located in the tendons of the masticatory muscles, in the TMJ capsule, in the mandibular and maxillary periosteum, in the periodontal membrane and the oral mucous membrane, all provide afferent discharges to motor neurone pools in the central nervous system where their combined facilitatory and inhibitory influences result in reflex coordination of muscle activity.

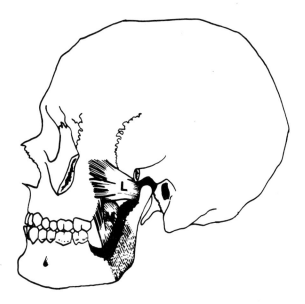

Figure 2.10 The pterygoid muscles: M medial pterygoid; L lateral pterygoid

Functional movement of the mandible

Protrusion of the mandible

Once the mandible is lowered sufficiently to clear the cusps of the teeth, the jaw can be moved forward. In so doing the condyles move down a slope along a path which is normally almost straight. The inclination of this path is different from the inclination of the bony part of the articular eminence since variations in thickness of the disc and the other soft tissue surfaces are involved.

The major muscle causing the forward movement of the mandible in the sagittal plane is the lower head of the lateral pterygoid muscle, although occasional irregular activity of the masseter and medial pterygoid muscles have been detected electromyographically. The posterior part of the temporal muscle and digastric muscle act as antagonists.

Retrusion of the mandible

Posterior sagittal translation is achieved by relaxation of the lower head of the lateral pterygoid muscle, while the superior head remains in tension, together with traction of the posterior fibres of the temporal muscle, which is the dominant muscle in this movement. The digastric muscle also assists in posterior translation, as well as the deep part of the masseter muscle.

Lateral movements of the mandible

During side movements (laterotrusion) and chewing, the jaw rotates about a vertical axis near the working condyle. The non-working condyle moves in protrusion/retrusion with the appropriate muscle activity on that side.

Habitual mouth opening and closing

Opening movements of the mandible are accomplished by the combined action of the lateral pterygoid muscle, together with the anterior belly of the digastric muscle which is active during rotation of the mandible.

Observations during elevation of the mandible show consistent activity in the temporal and masseter muscles and also in the medial pterygoid. There is also activity in the lateral pterygoid muscle, but this would not be related to the movement of the mandible, but rather to a stabilization of the condylar head during rotation.

Under normal resting conditions the mandible is in a relaxed position with a small inter-occlusal space between the teeth. On closure to the intercuspal position, the condyles mainly rotate on their discs. The inter-occlusal space is normally referred to as the freeway space. It has been shown that this postural position is partly under reflex muscle control and partly controlled by connective tissue elasticity. In clinical practice, establishing the postural position is difficult since a variety of factors can cause changes in reflex control of the muscles and thereby also the position of the mandible.

Condylar movements

During initial opening from centric occlusion the condyle will rotate on the disc and the jaw will move to the postural position. As the jaw opens further the disc begins to translate forward, whilst the condyle moves forward over the disc surface. The condyle translates forward about 8 mm on the disc and, together with the disc movement, there is translation forward of about 15 mm.

The condyle thus moves in a smooth curve passing over the various bands of the disc and pulling the soft tissues distal to the joint forward, stretching their posterior attachments.

During chewing the working side condyle moves slightly backwards, upwards and outwards and the non-working condyle moves forward, downwards and inwards. This lateral bodily movement of the mandible is referred to as the Bennett movement or side shift.

Further reading

de Bont L G M (1985) *Temporomandibular Joint. Articular Cartilage Structure and Function*. Van Denderen, Amsterdam
Klineberg I (1971) Structure and function of temporomandibular joint innervation. *Annals of the Royal College of Surgeons of England*, **49**, 268–288
Kopp S (1992) Diagnosis and nonsurgical treatment of the arthritides. Connective tissue aspects. In: *The Temporomandibular Joint. A Biological Basis for Clinical Practice* (eds B G Sarnat and D M Laskin). W B Saunders, pp. 357–359
McDevitt W E (1989) *Functional Anatomy of the Masticatory System*. Wright, London
McKay G S, Yemm R and Cadden S W (1992) The structure and function of the temporomandibular joint. *British Dental Journal*, **173**, 127–132
Meyenberg K, Kubik S and Palla S (1986) Relationship of the muscles of mastication to the articular disc of the temporomandibular joint. *Helvetica Odontologica Acta*, **30**, 815–834
Mohl N D, Zarb G A, Carlsson G E and Rugh J D (1988) *A Textbook of Occlusion*. Quintessence, Chicago
Sperber G H (1989) *Craniofacial Embryology*. Wright, London
Zarb G A and Carlsson G E (1979) *Temporomandibular Joint Function and Dysfunction*. Munksgaard, Copenhagen

3

Aetiology

It is generally agreed that the aetiology of symptoms of TMJ dysfunction is *multifactorial*. That is to say that several different factors acting alone or in varying combinations may be responsible. Various emotional and mechanical factors have been implicated. In some cases the emotional component is minimal while at other times it may be of prime importance. Common to all the mechanical factors is adverse loading or overloading of the tissues which may be as a result of a single event such as a blow to the face or be a consequence of repetitive minor trauma.

Aetiological factors may be described as being *predisposing*, *precipitating* or *perpetuating* although in practice such a distinction may be difficult to determine clinically.

Predisposing factors

It is reasonable to assume that various anatomical, physiological and biochemical factors predispose an individual to TMJ dysfunction, as may occur in genetic or inherited disorders. At present little is known about this. In addition, neurological, vascular, nutritional or metabolic disorders can affect the musculoskeletal tissues and predispose an individual to TMJ problems.

It is well recognized that certain individuals are susceptible to stress-related conditions and it has been shown that these individuals have a higher incidence of TMJ dysfunction than other individuals. Certain individuals show considerable tension in specific muscle groups under stress.

Precipitating factors

Stress–psychological factors

Chronic stress is an important aetiological factor in a variety of psychosomatic disorders such as peptic ulcer, chronic back pain and various skin disorders and it is also believed to play a crucial role in the aetiology of symptoms of TMJ dysfunction in many patients. Many TMJ dysfunction patients have psychological characteristics that make them more likely to experience emotional difficulties in dealing with stressful life events and among these are family bereavement, illness, divorce and moving house. Of a group of patients with TMJ dysfunction 78% had suffered an adverse life event such as family health problems, bereavement or marital difficulty prior to the onset of the pain. In addition 80% of the patients also complained of other stress-related disorders such as headaches, aches in the neck and back, dermatitis or pruritis, spastic colon and dysfunctional uterine bleeding (Feinmann and Harris, 1984).

The pathogenesis of the stress-related symptoms in TMJ dysfunction is believed to be related to increased autonomic activity causing increased facial muscle activity. Harris *et al.*, 1993 postulated that emotional stress can stimulate the release of neuropeptides which can induce a painful myositis capsulitis or synovitis. Stress is also associated with habitual tooth clenching and bruxism which can also produce symptoms of TMJ dysfunction.

Various neurotic conditions such as anxiety neurosis, minor stress disorders and post-traumatic stress syndrome are also associated with increased muscular activity and may be important aetiologic factors in TMJ dysfunction and recurrent headaches in patients with these psychological illnesses (Enoch and Jagger, 1994).

Bruxism

Bruxism may be defined as purposeless rhythmical, habitual tooth clenching or grinding movements which may occur either while awake or during sleep.

Habitual tooth pressing or clenching has been termed diurnal bruxism whilst tooth grinding, which usually occurs during sleep, has been called nocturnal bruxism.

PREVALENCE OF BRUXISM

The prevalence of bruxism is difficult to determine since the activity is performed subconsciously and questioning alone is therefore unreliable. Studies by questionnaire, however, have reported that approximately 15–20% of people are aware of bruxing or habitually clenching their teeth.

Bruxism is common in young children from the time the deciduous teeth erupt and it is found in all age groups in both dentate subjects and in those with artificial teeth.

AETIOLOGY OF BRUXISM

The aetiology of bruxism is uncertain, but several factors have been implicated:

Psychic stress. The relationship between emotional stress and bruxism has been demonstrated by the use of an electromyographic device which was worn when subjects were asleep.

Investigations have confirmed that stressful daytime situations, such as domestic quarrels, violent cinema films etc. evoke an immediate increase in muscular activity and that such stressful situations are found to be correlated with high levels of tooth grinding at night. Nocturnal bruxism is now considered to be a sleep disorder that is stress related.

Occlusal interferences. Premature occlusal contacts on closure of the mandible in the retruded contact position and balancing side interferences have been found to be relatively more frequent in bruxists. Clinical experience suggests that removal of these occlusal interferences can reduce bruxism and experimental bruxism has been produced in humans and animals by the introduction of occlusal prematurities.

Other factors. Bruxism can be induced in animals by stimulation of specific cortical areas of the brain. Certain cerebral injuries are known to cause bruxism and amongst children with cerebral palsy the incidence of bruxism is high.

Magnesium deficiency and other dietary factors are able to elicit muscular hyperactivity similar to that which takes place in bruxism, and muscular hyperactivity has been noted as a side-effect of medication with both amphetamines for weight reduction and levodopa for the treatment of Parkinson's disease. Genetic factors also play a role in the predisposition to bruxism since monozygotic twins have been shown to have a higher degree of similarity in the tooth facet pattern than dizygotic twins.

DIAGNOSIS OF BRUXISM

The diagnosis of bruxism is not always easily made because the activity is performed subconsciously and an individual is often unaware of the habit. Diagnostic features comprise the following:

● occlusal sounds during sleep—a positive diagnostic sign
● functional tooth surface wear, i.e. attrition facets
● periodontal changes described above
● masticatory muscle fatigue or pain, especially on waking

- masticatory muscle tenderness
- recurrent headaches
- fractured fillings or split teeth
- soreness of oral mucosa beneath dentures
- tenderness upon percussion of teeth
- mucosal ridging of tongue and cheeks.

EFFECT ON MASTICATORY MUSCLES AND TEMPOROMANDIBULAR JOINTS

Experimental clenching of the teeth leads to masticatory muscle fatigue and pain similar to that reported by patients suffering from TMJ dysfunction. These induced symptoms have been associated with an aseptic non-serous inflammation in the connective tissue component of the muscle. Prolonged static muscle tension is a common explanation of the aetiological mechanism of this inflammation and the subsequent pain. Overloading the articular tissues may result in a traumatic arthritis. Hypertrophy of masseter muscles may occur.

EFFECT ON TEETH

An early sign of bruxism is the presence of shiny facets on the functional surfaces of teeth or restorations in both centric and excursive/eccentric positions of the jaw. These facets fit together with matching facets in the opposing dentition. Further bruxism leads to a greater attrition of enamel, which occasionally flakes off. Cupping of exposed dentine can occur and in excessive tooth wear pulpal exposure may take place.

EFFECT ON PERIODONTAL TISSUES

Protective reaction by the periodontal tissues to compensate for heavy occlusal forces results in hypertrophy of periodontal tissues. Thickening of alveolar bone, exostosis formation, increased trabeculation of the alveolar process, a thickened periodontal membrane, consisting of heavy collagenous fibres, and increased periodontal fibre attachment to the cementum are observed.

Bruxism *per se* does not induce gingivitis or periodontal disease. However, in association with marginal periodontitis, occlusal trauma may lead to an accelerated destruction of the periodontal tissues and to an increase in alveolar bone loss. Pain or tenderness in the supporting soft tissues of the teeth may be a sign of bruxism.

Oral habits—parafunction

A common finding in patients with TMJ dysfunction is that they unconsciously perform purposeless jaw movements which results in increased physical load on the masticatory muscles. A typical observation is that there is a finger nail-biting habit. Since this necessitates protrusion and elevation of the jaw, often eccentrically, it is not surprising to find that the lateral pterygoid and masseter muscles become tender following prolonged excitation.

Other habits such as chewing pencils, biting the cheeks or chewing gum may lead to a similar response. Occupational conditions such as biting thread in textile factories may also cause problems.

Trauma

Trauma, such as a blow to the jaw, may lead to inflammation and tissue damage. The musculature is usually not damaged permanently and after a period of rest, full recovery occurs. Perpetuating factors such as bruxism may delay healing. The joint is different in this respect and there may be tearing or rupture of the posterior attachment of the disc. In many cases rest will lead to recovery and/ or healing, but in other instances the damage can lead to permanent damage or disc displacement and the patient may experience persistent symptoms.

The term *microtrauma* has been used to describe the effect of repetitive-strain type injuries that also might damage the temporomandibular joint or muscles of mastication. Occlusal interference, bruxism, and nail biting are examples of activities that might produce microtrauma.

Some patients who have suffered cervical hyperextension/ hyperflexion ('whiplash') injury complain of the onset symptoms of TMJ dysfunction in addition to other neck and head symptoms. The pathogenesis of the TMJ symptoms is uncertain. There are three possible mechanisms:

- direct traumatic damage to TMJs and muscles of mastication
- referred symptoms from damaged cervical nerves to the trigeminal distribution
- post-traumatic stress syndrome producing hyperactivity of muscles of mastication.

Late symptoms following condylar fractures are rarely encountered in children because the capacity of the joints to undergo remodelling but in adults symptoms may persist after treatment. Late symptoms may also appear in adults on the uninjured side due to alteration in mandibular function. Fibrous or bony ankylosis may occasionally occur after a fracture with associated intra-articular bleeding, particularly if treatment includes prolonged mandibular immobilization. Symptoms of dysfunction are particularly common after unilateral subcondylar fracture with significant fracture displacement.

Occlusal abnormalities

The role of malocclusion and occlusal interferences in the aetiology of TMJ dysfunction has been the subject of much debate and controversy. A complicating factor is that TMJ problems may themselves be responsible for causing occlusal interferences. Specific occlusal factors have not been shown to have a predictive value in determining whether TMJ dysfunction will develop. A balanced view would be that on some occasions, occlusal irregularities may be important contributing factors but that further scientifically controlled, longitudinal studies are needed to provide more reliable information concerning the relationship between occlusion and TMJ dysfunction.

The following occlusal factors are believed to be of importance.

OCCLUSAL DEFICIENCIES

Although the peak incidence of pain is in the third and fourth decades, it is also often experienced by older adults who have suffered the loss of posterior teeth. A common finding is that TMJ dysfunction occurs when there is loss of molar support, which forces the patient to chew on the anterior teeth rather than to use them purely for incision. This necessitates continual abnormal use of the masticatory muscles with consequent risk of overuse and pain.

Unilateral loss of natural teeth will result in unilateral mastication. This will require increased action by the ipsilateral lateral pterygoid and the contralateral masseter muscle. Increased loading of the TMJ resulting from loss of posterior support is believed to be an important aetiological factor and restoration of the occlusion for this group of patients presenting with TMJ pain is recommended. Tooth loss may act as a precipitating or perpetuating factor and whilst many patients who have an inadequate occlusion do not develop TMJ dysfunction, those with some other factor already present will be subjected to a higher risk of its development.

INTERFERENCES

It is a common clinical observation that the introduction of an occlusal interference, e.g. by an inadequately contoured restoration, may lead to TMJ dysfunction. Following extraction of teeth, drifting and tilting of the remaining teeth in the arch can take place. Occlusal interferences can be created which cause deviation of the lower jaw into an eccentric position, after and to tension or pain in the musculature. In some individuals slight interferences can lead to TMJ problems, whilst in others gross abnormalities exist with no problems. The basic parameters which are considered essential to create an occlusion which will not cause dysfunction are described in detail in Chapter 4.

VERTICAL DIMENSION

Alteration of the occlusal vertical dimension may produce symptoms of dysfunction. Costen's original contention that 'overclosure' was the pertinent cause of TMJ symptoms has been discounted, but it is widely considered that long-standing overclosure may be an aetiological factor. Whilst young tissues may adapt to fairly large alterations in vertical dimension, sudden increase in occlusal vertical dimension, particularly in an elderly edentulous patient with long-standing overclosure, can also precipitate dysfunction.

INCISOR RELATIONSHIP

It has been suggested that undue forces are placed on the TMJs and masticatory muscles as a consequence of an unfavourable incisor relationship. Studies to date suggest that factors such as increased overjet and overbite and negative overbite (anterior open-bite) are likely to be predisposing factors rather than initiating factors in the production of symptoms of TMJ dysfunction.

Perpetuating factors

These may be related to any combination of predisposing or precipitating factors. It is believe that psychoimmunological changes may result from chronic distress and pain. These may act as perpetuating factors.

Chronic pain conditions, including chronic facial pain, are commonly associated with clinical depression. As the duration of a pain continues it becomes centralized and its clinical characteristics merged with psychological. It becomes impossible to tell whether the depression is an aetiological factor or a consequence of that pain.

Further reading

Carlsson G E and Droukas B (1984) Dental occlusion and the health of the masticatory system. *Journal of Craniomandibular Practice*, **2**, 141–147

Dworkin S F and Burgess J A (1987) Orofacial pain of psychogenic origin: current concepts and classification. *Journal of the American Dental Association*, **115**, 565–571

Feinmann C and Harris M (1984) Psychogenic pain Part 1: The clinical presentation. *British Dental Journal*, **156**, 165–168

Mohl N D, Zarb G A, Carlsson G E and Rugh J D (1988) Occlusal parafunction. In: *A Textbook of Occlusion*. Quintessence, Chicago, pp. 249–261

Mohl N D (1993) Reliability and validity of diagnostic modalities for temporomandibular disorders. *Advances in Dental Research*, **7**, 113–119

Rugh J D and Solberg W K (1979) Psychological implications in temporomandibular pain and dysfunction. In: *TMJ—Function and Dysfunction* (Zarb G and Carlsson G E, eds). Munksgaard, Copenhagen

Rugh J D (1987) Psychological components of pain. *Dental Clinics of North America*, **1**, 579–594

Rugh J D, Woods B J and Dahlström I (1993) Temporomandibular disorders. Assessment of psychological factors. *Advances in Dental Research*, **7**, 127–136

Yemm R (1976) Neurophysiological studies of temporomandibular joint dysfunction. *Oral Science Reviews*, **7**, 31–53

4

History and examination

History

In order to diagnose correctly a temporomandibular disorder a complete history and examination is usually needed. The signs and symptoms of TMJ dysfunction are sometimes sufficiently distinctive to identify readily the problem. At other times the diagnosis may be much harder to determine particularly if there is a chronic diffuse pain of a sort that may be produced by a variety of pathologies. The history of the presenting complaint(s) as well as past dental and medical history are all important parts of the clinical investigation.

It is important to semi-structure the taking of the history because patients can introduce many irrelevant or diversionary details even though they are trying to be helpful. A suggested structure is:

1. List presenting complaints
2. Description of presenting complaint(s)
3. History of complaints
4. Aetiological factors—mechanical
                                  emotional
5. Dental history
6. Medical history including—musculoskeletal disorders
                                  stress-related disorders
                                  recurrent headaches

A list of the patient's presenting orofacial symptoms should be made and a clear description and history of those complaints obtained.

Most dentists are very familiar with the process of detailed investigation of *pain* of uncertain origin and are aware of the importance of a logical and comprehensive history that includes the following:

Location and radiation
Nature (sharp, dull, throbbing, etc.)
Severity
Duration

Frequency
Exacerbating/relieving factors

The patient should be asked to describe TMJ *sounds* and to provide details of *restriction of mandibular movement* as well as associated symptoms such as vertigo or ear symptoms described in Chapter 1.

Potential *aetiological factors* must be identified. Patients should be asked whether any trauma to the mouth or face precipitated symptoms. Patients often deny habitually clenching the teeth or nocturnal bruxing but on a later occasion might report that he/she has become aware of the problem either by personal observation or by being told by close relatives.

Patients should be asked specifically about anxiety, depression and stressful life events. The use of screening inventories or questionnaires to detect psycho-pathology has been recommended. Lengthy comprehensive inventories are available but require the skills of a trained psychologist. Further developmental work is necessary in this area in order to provide dentists with a convenient valid screening device to detect psychological/psychiatric disorders in patients with facial pain.

The *medical history* should include questions relating to other muscle and joint problems. A conventional medical history should be obtained but must include questions relating to recurrent headaches, other muscle and joint problems and stress-related disorders.

Having obtained the history it is useful to relate a concise summary to the patient so that any inaccuracies or omissions can be corrected. This also gives the patient an opportunity to discuss any particular worries before starting the examination.

Examination

The muscles

Examination of masticatory muscles is principally by palpation. Palpation is not a difficult technique but needs a good knowledge of anatomy as well as a degree of practice.

Palpation is performed by the finger-tips, starting with a light but gradually increasing pressure. The pressure should not hurt the patient, who should be observed for pain reflexes (twitching of the eyelids). The degree of the response to the palpatory pressure is determined. Bilateral palpation is performed and the patient is asked to report any difference in sensation between right and left sides, rather than whether it hurts. It is also sometimes possible to detect small, painful fibrous nodules in affected muscles.

One should be cautious in the interpretation of the results of palpation. There are areas in the masticatory system that are more sensitive than others to palpation and therefore more likely to elicit a stronger response. This is true especially for palpation in the region of the lateral pterygoid muscle. The examiner should try to avoid too great a pressure, which can provoke pain by tissue compression. One way to check the palpatory findings (besides the aforementioned comparison between right and left sides) is to determine how the muscle reacts when it is activated. Contraction of the muscle will elicit pain if it is affected.

PROCEDURE

The palpation of the muscles of mastication and associated structures should follow a set procedure, preferably starting with the extraoral and followed by the intraoral palpation.

EXTRAORAL PALPATION (Figs 4.1–4.8)

● Lateral palpation of the TMJs.
● Posterior palpation of the temporomandibular joints through the external auditory meatus.
● The anterior and posterior parts of the origin and belly of the temporalis muscle.
● The superficial portion of the masseter muscle.
● The insertion of the medial pterygoid (angle of the mandible).
● The anterior and posterior belly of the digastric muscle.
● The sternocleidomastoid muscle.
● The muscles of the neck.
● The trapezius muscle.

INTRAORAL PALPATION (Figs 4.9–4.13)

● The superficial and deep portions of the masseter muscle (bidigital palpation).
● The insertion of the temporalis muscle on the coronoid process.
● The lateral pterygoid muscle behind the maxillary tuberosity.
● The medial pterygoid muscle.
● The muscles of the floor of the mouth (bidigital palpation).

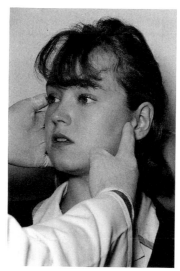

Figure 4.1 Lateral palpation of the TMJ

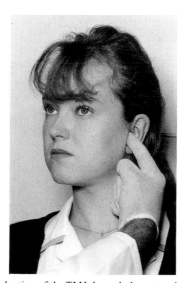

Figure 4.2 Posterior palpation of the TMJ through the external auditory meatus

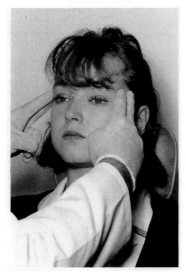

Figure 4.3 Palpation of anterior part of the origin and belly of the temporalis muscle

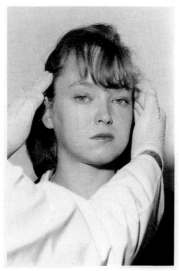

Figure 4.4 Palpation of posterior part of the origin and belly of the temporalis muscle

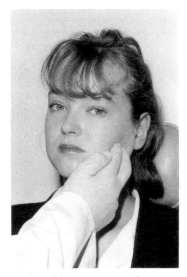

Figure 4.5 The superficial portion of the masseter muscle

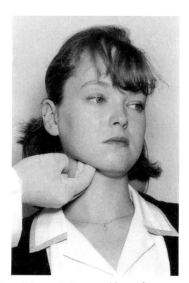

Figure 4.6 The insertion of the medial pterygoid muscle

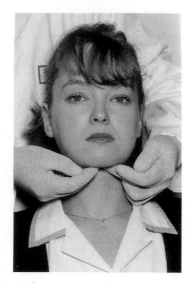

Figure 4.7 The digastric muscle

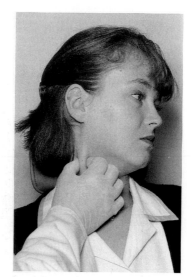

Figure 4.8 The sternocleidomastoid muscle

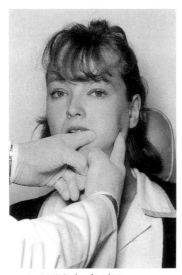

Figure 4.9 The masseter muscle, bidigital palpation

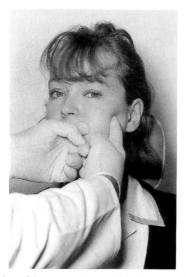

Figure 4.10 The insertion of the temporalis muscle to the coronoid process

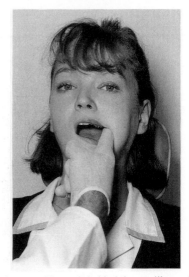

Figure 4.11 The lateral pterygoid muscle behind the maxillary tuberosity

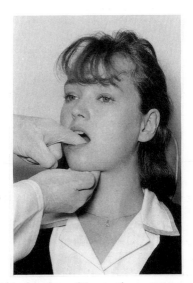

Figure 4.12 The muscles of the floor of the mouth

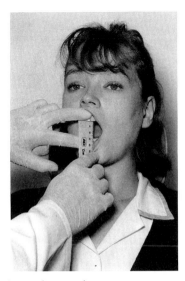

Figure 4.13 Measuring the opening capacity

THE MASSETER MUSCLE

The whole superficial portion is easily accessible, whereas the deep portion can be reached extraorally at the origin below the zygomatic arch only. The extraoral palpation can be supplemented by bidigital palpation, whereby the relaxed muscle is embraced between fingers. The anterior border of the muscle can be easily palpated from the origin down to the insertion. If the patient is requested to clench his teeth, the difference between relaxed and contracted muscle can be felt easily and tenderness in a specific part of the muscle readily identified.

THE TEMPORALIS MUSCLE

This muscle too can be palpated both extra- and intraorally. The examination of the origin and belly should include the anterior third as well as the posterior two-thirds. The origin of the temporalis muscle can be felt beneath the scalp at the level of the superior temporal line when the patient is clenching his teeth. The belly of the temporalis muscle is accessible for palpation in the temporal fossa, which is located just above the zygomatic arch and just behind the lateral corner of the eye. The insertion can be palpated intraorally by letting the patient open his mouth to move the coronoid process forward–downward below the zygomatic arch. The anterior border of the ramus is followed upwards bilaterally by the index fingers to reach the insertion area on the upper, inner surface of the coronoid process.

THE MEDIAL PTERYGOID MUSCLE

This muscle is difficult to reach, especially at its origin. However, the muscle can be palpated almost in its entire length by carefully moving the index finger along the anterior surface of the ramus. The patient often finds this procedure disagreeable and a vomiting reflex may sometimes be provoked. One way to avoid this is to instruct the patient to take a deep breath and hold it until the palpation is finished. The index finger is moved under pressure from the pterygoid notch region down along the inside of the ramus to the region of insertion on the interior side of the mandibular angle. At the angle of the mandible supplemental bidigital palpation can be performed by putting fingers of the other hand against the outer border of the mandible. At the same time the head can be moved forward, downward and laterally in order to determine the degree of tenderness more precisely. If palpation produces problems for the patient, extraoral palpation of the insertion of the muscle at the angle of the mandible will suffice. It should be noted, however, that other tender structures can be present in this region, e.g. lymph nodes.

THE LATERAL PTERYGOID MUSCLE

The inferior belly only can be compressed by palpation. The palpation is performed with the tip of the index or little finger, which is moved behind the maxillary tuberosity in a medio-postero-superior direction where it is possible to compress the muscle. This region is normally sensitive in most individuals and it is important to compare the response of the right and left side.

DIGASTRIC MUSCLE

This muscle is palpated bilaterally by the index or little fingers placed between the posterior border of the mandibular ramus and the mastoid process. The fingers are gently pressed in a medial direction where the muscle belly can be felt, especially if the patient swallows or performs a retrusive movement of the mandible.

THE MUSCLES OF THE FLOOR OF THE MOUTH

These muscles are palpated intraorally by the index and middle fingers of one hand while the mandible is stabilized by the other hand.

THE STERNOCLEIDOMASTOID MUSCLE

This muscle has two origins, one on the manubrium of the sternum, the other on the medial part of the clavicle. The belly is easily seen if the patient bends his head antero-inferiorly and to the contralateral side. The muscle should not be compressed inwards, but lifted out and palpated from the sides due to the presence of the carotid sinus and the risk of a drop in blood pressure. Tender areas are often found where the two bellies of the muscle converge and in the insertion of the muscle on the posterior part of the mastoid process.

THE TRAPEZIUS MUSCLE

The parts around the shoulder are palpated up to the insertion on the back of the head. The patient is then asked to raise his shoulder and, if possible, twist it a little forward towards his chest. The musculature is then fairly well relaxed. Where contraction of the muscle is of long duration, the ability to twist the neck is often impaired.

Temporomandibular joint

The clinical examination of the TMJ should comprise inspection, palpation and auscultation.

INSPECTION

Inspection of the joint area should be performed with respect to redness and swelling, which can indicate acute inflammatory conditions of the joint (rheumatoid arthritis, septic arthritis, traumatic arthritis) and scarring which may indicate past local diseases and operative procedures. Swelling of the TMJ is not restricted to the area just outside the joint, but extends down to the insertion of the capsule on the condylar neck.

PALPATION

Palpation of the TMJs is performed bilaterally and will provide information about the movement capacity of the joint, irregularities of the joint movements, clicking and crepitation as well as a degree of joint tenderness.

The movement capacity of the condyles is estimated by careful bilateral palpation of the joints by the finger-tips. The patient is asked to perform mandibular opening and closing movements during this procedure. Attempt is thereby made to estimate the range of condylar movement and to detect any differences between right and left sides.

Irregularities of the condylar movement can be palpated as sudden interruption in the smooth movement of the joint and are often associated with a clicking sound.

Crepitation of the joint can be felt as a grating sensation by the finger-tips during mandibular movements. The patient should perform opening and closing movements as well as protrusive and laterotrusive movements and the chin observed for deviation during the opening and protrusion movements.

The degree of tenderness is judged by bilateral palpation from the lateral prominences of the condyles, and posteriorly via the external auditory meatus. The examiner during this procedure should stand or sit in front of the patient who is asked to keep the mandible in a relaxed position. If the mandible is moved during palpation, pain may be provoked by the movement itself rather than by the palpatory pressure. It is always difficult to estimate the degree of palpatory tenderness, but a difference in tenderness between right and left sides reported by the patient or visible pain reflexes should be noted. If pain is evoked only by lateral palpation of the joint it may originate from the musculature just in front of the joint. On the other hand, if pain is evoked by palpation posteriorly as well as laterally the joint tissues proper are probably involved.

AUSCULTATION

Auscultation can reveal the presence and character of joint sounds, and where in the movement pattern the sounds occur. From a diagnostic point of view it is important to differentiate between clicks and crepitation. Clicks are regarded as being caused by muscular incoordination, deviation in articular form or disc displacement, whereas crepitation indicates the presence of pathologic irregularity of the joint surfaces. The most sensitive way to detect joint sounds is to use a stethoscope which should be placed on the zygomatic process rather than on the joint to avoid disturbing sounds caused by joint movement.

Examination of the mandibular movements

Mandibular movement is often affected. An examination of the mandibular movements is therefore essential in a functional evaluation of the TMJs and muscles of mastication.

THE OPENING MOVEMENTS

The clinical examination of the vertical movement can be facilitated by a pencil marking of the midline on an incisor, or on the chin or by putting tooth picks between the central incisors in both upper and lower jaw. Standing in front of the patient it is easy to see how the markings are moved in relation to each other and to notice lateral deviations during the opening and closing movements. The size of the deviation is estimated and its location on the path of movement as well as associated pain, joint sounds, locking or asymmetry. A simple drawing of the path of movement can be made in the notes, where the type of deviation is described and the direction of the movement is indicated by arrows. Deviation during the protrusive movement can be recorded in the same way.

THE MOVEMENT CAPACITY

The degree of disturbance of the stomatognathic system is assessed by measurement of the mandibular maximal movement capacity. Acute pain in the TMJ area or the masticatory musculature almost always causes a restriction of mandibular movement.

Exact upper and lower limits of normal mobility of the mandible are difficult to state since there are great individual variations, but the lower limit of maximal opening is usually in the region of 40 mm for adults.

Measurement of mandibular mobility can be made by a millimetre ruler. The edge of the ruler is placed on the edges of the lower central incisors and the distance to the incisal edges of the upper central incisors is estimated to the nearest millimetre when the patient opens his mouth as much as possible (Fig. 4.13). The value is called the maximal voluntary interincisor distance. The maximal opening capacity is achieved when the vertical incisor overbite is added.

In order to facilitate the measurement of the laterotrusive and protrusive movements a vertical line is marked with a pencil on the facial surfaces of the central incisors and on the buccal surfaces of an occluding pair of premolars when the mandible is in centric occlusion (CO). The distance between markings can then be

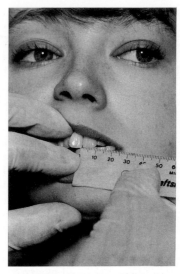

Figure 4.14 Measuring lateral movement capacity

measured when the patient performs maximal, active movements in the respective directions (Fig. 4.14).

The movement between the centric relation (CR) and centric occlusion (CO) is preferably estimated when the occlusion is examined. In epidemiological studies the distance between CO and CR has been commonly found to be slightly less than 1 mm.

PAIN ON MOVEMENT

An examination of the movements of the mandible should also include questions about pain during the movements as well as observation of pain reflexes. The patient is asked about location, character and intensity of the pain. One movement is examined at a time and an attempt is made to decide if the pain originates in the muscles or joints. The patient can seldom decide himself if the pain is coming from the muscles or the joints and even relatively distant muscle pain can be located to the joint proper (referred pain). To facilitate this judgement both active and passive movements are examined. An active movement is performed by the patient himself by own muscle activity. Passive movement is performed by the examiner guiding the mandible, while the patient is passive and as relaxed as possible. If the pain originates in the muscles, as a rule, the active movement is more restricted than the passive. On the other hand, if active and passive movements are approximately the same, the pain probably originates in the joint. When the joints are affected the patient often experiences pain during most of the extensive mandibular movements, while muscular pain is usually provoked during movements when the affected muscles are principally engaged (e.g. an affected left lateral pterygoid muscle hurts on laterotrusion to the right, but usually not on laterotrusion to the left). Movements against resistance (isometric muscle contraction) can be instituted to accentuate diffuse pain responses, since the active muscles are forced to contract forcefully whilst maintaining the same length. The strength of the muscles can be roughly estimated at the same time.

POSTURAL POSITION OF THE MANDIBLE AND FREEWAY SPACE

The freeway space can be defined as the distance between the occlusal surfaces when the mandible assumes its postural position. The postural position is not a definite position, but a position that is subjected to constant changes in the vertical as well as horizontal plane. Factors which influence the postural position and thus the size of the freeway space are age, health, body and head posture, breathing, mental and neuromuscular tensions, and the dental condition of the individual (degree of dental attrition, tooth losses and prosthetic appliances). Furthermore the method used to determine the postural position also influences the size of the freeway space.

The following methods can be recommended for use in the determination: relaxation, swallowing and sounding of the letter 'm'. It should be noted that the sounding of 'm' produces a significantly greater freeway space than the other two methods. The measurement of the freeway space can be performed clinically using a Willis gauge or calipers. The accuracy of determination of resting position is not of a high order.

Examination of the occlusion

An examination of the occlusion should include examination of the individual teeth, the morphology of the dental arches, and an estimation of function. One of the most important aspects of the functional examination is to examine the tooth contacts during chewing and articulation. The examination should be performed according to a systematic scheme and the different occlusal positions and articulatory movements should be thoroughly differentiated in order to detect occlusal interferences. The most important mandibular reference positions can be defined as follows.

CENTRIC RELATION (CR)

Centric relation is the relationship between mandible and maxilla when the condyles are most posteriorly and superiorly in the glenoid fossae.

RETRUDED CONTACT POSITION (RCP)

Retruded contact position is the position of the mandible when first tooth contact is made when closing on the terminal hinge axis.

CENTRIC OCCLUSION (CO)

Centric occlusion is the position of the mandible where the maximal occlusal contact occurs. Synonym: intercuspal position.

POSTURAL POSITION (REST POSITION)

Postural position is the position of the mandible when the individual is standing or sitting upright in a relaxed position freely, is looking straight forward and when the masticatory muscles have minimal activity.

INTERFERENCE

Interference is the first contact between a tooth and its antagonist or a part of a prosthesis, which prevents contact in other parts of the occlusion. Synonym: premature contact.

Centric relation is the most important reference position of the mandible for the following reasons:

- It is the most constant and reproducible position of the mandible and therefore more reliable than non-hinge positions.
- It permits a comparison of the positions of the midline of the mandible in postural position and other positions.
- It is a position on a simple movement path, the terminal hinge movement, and is therefore suitable to use for mounting casts of the lower jaw in the articulator.

A functional examination of the occlusion includes observation of the tooth contacts in RCP and CO during gliding between these positions and during articulation (contact movements). The appropriate technique for the different phases of the functional examination of the occlusion is described as follows.

Relationship between centric relation and centric occlusion
Several techniques have been recommended to reach and examine
CR. One recommended technique is as follows:

- The patient should be comfortably lying in a chair with good
  head support. Try to get the patient relaxed.
- Hold the patient's chin with your thumb against the lower
  alveolar ridge and your index finger below the chin. Ask the
  patient to open the mouth and relax as much as possible. The
  examiner should guide and move the mandible up and down in
  rotary movements and the patient should avoid making any
  resistance against this movement.
- Move the mandible up and down without tooth contact and
  push at the same time the mandible backwards with a slight pressure. Repeat this procedure until it is relaxed and reproducible.
- After the hinge movement has been practised the examiner's
  thumb is placed on the facial surfaces of the lower incisors
  and the mandible is pressed backwards with a slight, constant
  pressure and is then guided to the first contact with the upper
  jaw.
  Once the retruded contact position has been achieved, it is
  usually easy to repeat the procedure for a more thorough
  examination of the slide between CR and CO. This part of the
  clinical examination is supplemented by the patient's own
  observations and should consist of the following:

(a) The contact relationships in the retruded position.
(b) The presence of lateral displacement of the mandible during
    the slide between CR and CO.
(c) Insufficient balance during the slide between CR and CO
    (unilateral contacts).
(d) A distance greater than 2 mm between CR and CO.

The patient can also frequently, without difficulty, tell whether
there is unilateral or bilateral contact or tell which teeth make
the first occlusal contact. When judging the movement between
RCP and CO, its direction, balance and extent are observed.
The examination is facilitated if the jaw relationship in CO is
recorded by marking the teeth in the midline as well as in the
premolar area. Special consideration is given to the movement
between RCP and CO and whether it is associated with a lateral
displacement of the mandible.

- In order to refine the diagnostic procedure and to define the
  contact relationships in the RCP and to mark the exact position
  of interferences on the occlusal surfaces, different indicators are
  used.

OCCLUSAL RECORDING

Articulating paper has disadvantages in that it may also mark tooth surfaces which have no or very light contact. Ribbons provide more selective information.

The most distinct markings, however, are obtained by occlusal foil (Gebruder Hanel Medizinal, Nurtingen), which is very thin (8 μm) and preferably is used double to obtain markings in both upper and lower jaw at the same time. There are several other types of occlusal indicators on the market including coloured spray and occlusal wax (Fig. 4.15).

INTERCUSPAL POSITION

Centric occlusion (CO) can be judged in many ways, e.g. by direct inspection, by foil or wax indices, casts fitted by hand or mounted on an articulator. It should be stressed, however, that an examination of CO *per se*, gives no information about the functional state of the occlusion.

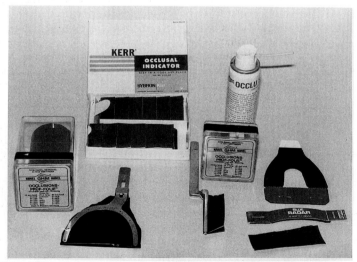

Figure 4.15 Articulating paper, ribbons, occlusal foil, occlusal wax and occlusal sprays

ARTICULATION

The examination of the articulation includes an appraisal of the character of the contact movements: lateral, medial and protrusive and combinations of these movements. The relationship between facets on the working and non-working sides is important.

The examination is carried out by:

(a) Letting the patient make slow, laterotrusive movement one side at a time, at first without tooth contact and then sliding movements with contact. The articulation contacts are carefully examined on both the working and non-working side.
(b) Guiding the mandible in a posterior (terminal) laterotrusive movement starting in CR and examining the articulation as above (a). This procedure is easiest performed on an articulator, but a comparison with the condition in the mouth should always be made.
(c) Letting the patient protrude habitually as well as in a controlled, 'straight' sagittal direction.

One should judge if the sliding movements are even and harmonious or whether they are uneven or disturbed by tooth locking. The preference by the patient for some movements should be observed, as well as difficulties in performing others and the reason for this ascertained. It is very important to differentiate the movements when examining the articulation. The number of contacts on the laterotrusive or working side is probably less important for the function of the masticatory system than a smooth and even movement. In a canine protected occlusion the teeth should separate smoothly, leaving only the canines in contact. When examining the mediotrusive or non-working side, attention is focused on the presence of mediotrusive- or non-working interferences, i.e. contacts on the non-working side, which result in loss of contact on the working side.

Such interferences have been thought to cause disturbances in the coordination of muscles and to evoke bruxism. They can be discovered by direct inspection, or by use of occlusal foil, thin paper strips, or wax indices.

One of the most important aspects of the examination of the occlusion is thus to discover interferences. The following are considered most important:

● Interferences which displace the mandible laterally during the slide between CR and CO.
● Balancing interferences.
● Instability of CO (loss of tooth contact).

TOOTH MOBILITY AND OCCLUSION

Premature contacts in the habitual closing path are best discovered by pressing the finger-tips lightly against the facial surfaces of the teeth during light closing movements. By careful inspection of each tooth during closing and during laterotrusive as well as protrusive movements, tooth mobility can be assessed. The exact position of the premature contact can be revealed with an indicator of foil, wax, or paper. It must be stressed, however, that although an increased tooth mobility often is a consequence of 'traumatic occlusion', a careful periodontal examination is essential.

ATTRITION FACETS

The examination of occlusion should also include a thorough inspection of the occlusal surfaces in order to find atypically located attrition facets indicating tooth clenching or grinding. The form and position of the facets may give information about the position and the movements of parafunction. It must be remembered, however, that discovered facets may have been produced long ago and do not necessarily indicate parafunctional activity at present. In order to clarify whether such facets are used in clenching/grinding and contribute to the symptoms of the patient, a so-called provocation test can be performed. This means that the patient is asked to keep his teeth clenched for about 1 minute in a suspected bruxing position. If this test provokes pain an objective of treatment is to prevent grinding/clenching in this position.

MORPHOLOGY OF OCCLUSION

Deviation in form, size and position of the teeth and dental arches that can elicit functional disturbances of the occlusion must also be considered. Mesially tipped second or third mandibular molars (following extraction of the first molar), over erupted teeth (following extraction of the antagonist), and teeth erupted outside the dental arches often disturb the articulation and cause unharmonious mandibular movements. Pathological conditions of the gingivae, periodontium and bone must be noted since they sometimes give rise to symptoms of pain and dysfunction.

Distemata should be investigated to establish if they have developed lately as a consequence of tooth migration.

OCCLUSION OF COMPLETE DENTURES

The occlusion of complete dentures cannot be judged outside the mouth. Despite a stable intercuspal position, the occlusion of the dentures may be wrong. It is not sufficient to examine the habitual closing path since the dentures and the mandible may be displaced into an incorrect intercuspal position. The appraisal must be made while keeping the denture in its proper location on the supporting tissues. The same rules, then, apply for the occlusion of complete dentures as for the natural dentition, except for balancing the denture in contact movements. Symptoms from the masticatory muscles and the TMJ and recurrent irritation to the supporting mucosa in patients with complete dentures can be caused by large differences between RCP and CO and by a deficient occlusal stability in CO. The treatment of choice is occlusal adjustment, which can be made temporarily by putting acrylic resin on the occlusal surfaces of the lower denture. This procedure is often combined with relining of the denture bases. A more permanent stabilization of the occlusion can be achieved by remounting using records taken in the CR combined with selective grinding or by making new dentures.

A short routine examination (screening)

The clinical examination described above need not be performed in full for all patients. A limited form of examination should, however, be performed for every new patient and for patients coming for review appointments.

A short functional examination of the stomatognathic system should include the following aspects:

- Palpation of TMJs and masticatory muscles (in particular the superficial portion of the masseter muscle, the anterior part of the origin of the temporalis muscle and insertion of the temporalis muscle on the coronoid process) in order to detect tenderness, pain and joint sounds.
- The mandibular mobility, vertical as well as horizontal movements with and without tooth contact, the presence of jerky movements and joint sounds.
- Occlusion and articulation with respect to the relation between CR and CO, the presence of interferences and increased tooth mobility.
- The morphology of the teeth and the dental arches with special reference to the number of occluding teeth, attrition facets, tipping, extrusion (supraposition) and development of diastema.

After some practice this simple functional examination, supplemented with a few questions about difficulties in opening the mouth and chewing, and recurrent headaches takes only about 2 minutes to perform.

Radiographic examination

Conventional intraoral radiographs may be necessary to exclude dental disease as the cause of a facial pain. Radiographs of the joint in both closed and open positions will establish if bony pathology is present. Suitable views include orthopantomographs and transcranial views. The transcranial views provide slightly superior visualization of joint surface irregularities commonly seen in degenerative changes. Dental practitioners are, however, more familiar with panoral radiographs, whereas transcranial views require the use of an extraoral cassette. Computed tomography (CT) provides optimum views of the joint surface but dosage is high.

The plain radiographic views described above can detect bony pathology but provide no information regarding soft tissue changes or disc displacement. For this the highly specialized techniques of arthrography or magnetic resonance imaging (MRI) are required.

Arthrography is an invasive technique in which a radio-opaque contrast medium is injected into either or both joint compartments. The lower compartment alone is usually chosen. Tomography recorded on a video camera can enable the movement of the condyle relative to the disc to be observed and the presence of the disc perforations to be detected. Intermittent freeze-frame fluoroscopy for needle placement and viewing reduces patient radiation exposure.

MRI is an expensive technique that produces superb images that require expert interpretation. It allows static visualization of hard and soft tissue but does not provide information about articular disc or posterior disc attachment perforations.

Radiographic assessment of a patient with symptoms of TMJ dysfunction usually involves a preliminary screening view, usually a panoral. If information is required about the presence of internal derangements, disc perforations and about function then arthrography is necessary. CT can provide detailed information regarding bony surfaces and CT also best defines joint spaces.

Direct visualization of articular tissue may be obtained by arthroscopy. This is also a highly specialized technique which is sometimes used to supplement radiographic investigation. It may be combined with articular irrigation with saline in a procedure termed lysis and lavage. A fine gauge arthroscope is introduced into the joint space. It has been recommended that this procedure be considered before more extensive surgery since it has been reported on occasions to lessen joint pain and to increase joint function.

Interpretation of arthroscopic images is difficult and arthroscopic diagnosis and treatment are still the subjects of investigation.

Further reading

Clark G T, Delcano R E and Goulet J-P (1993) The utility and validity of current diagnostic procedures for defining temporomandibular disorder patients. *Advances in Dental Research*, **7**, 97–112

Klineberg I (1991) *Occlusion: Principles and Assessment*. Wright, Oxford

McNeill C (ed) (1993) *Temporomandibular Disorders. Guidelines for Classification Assessment and Management* (2nd edn). The American Academy of Orofacial Pain. Quintessence, Chicago

Mohl N D, McCall W D, Lund J P and Plesh O (1990) Devices for the diagnosis and treatment of temporomandibular disorders. Part I: Introduction, scientific evidence, and jaw tracking. *Journal of Prosthetic Dentistry*, **63**, 198–201

Westesson P-L (1993) Reliability and validity of imaging diagnosis of temporomandibular joint disorder. *Advances in Dental Research*, **7**, 137–151

Wise M D (1986) *Occlusion and Restorative Dentistry for the General Practitioner* (2nd edn). British Dental Journal, London

5

Diagnosis and differential diagnosis

The diagnosis of facial pain must always be based upon a thorough history, examination and appropriate use of special investigations. The signs and symptoms of TMJ dysfunction are often sufficiently distinctive to readily identify the problem. The diagnosis of facial pain may be difficult, however, because it may represent the early stages of many diseases. A good knowledge of conditions having similar signs and symptoms is therefore necessary.

It is useful to relate the temporomandibular disorders to the classification of headache and orofacial pain devised by the International Headache Society (Cephalalgia, 1988) in order to appreciate the diverse nature of conditions associated with facial pain. Category 11 of this classification has been modified by the American Academy of Orofacial Pain (Appendix 1). Categories 11.7, temporomandibular disorders, and 11.8, masticatory muscle disorders, are of particular relevance. The distinctions between many of the non-specific articular and muscular conditions described in 11.7 and 11.8 are still the subject of investigation and the classification is subject to further revision (Dworkin and Le Resche, 1992) and has therefore not been used in this book. The relatively non-specific muscle and joint problems such as myositis, capsulitis and fibromyalgia are included in this text under the term TMJ dysfunction. This is a synonym for TMJ dysfunction syndrome and arthromyalgia. Anterior disc displacements are also included in this descriptive term.

Conditions affecting the TMJ and muscles of mastication are described below. Important conditions that may cause diagnostic confusion are described later in this chapter.

Disorders of TMJ and muscles of mastication

- TMJ dysfunction
- TMJ dislocation

- Arthritis
  osteoarthritis
  primary arthritis
- Ankylosis
- Neoplasia
- Congenital and developmental disorders.

TMJ dysfunction

The signs and symptoms associated with TMJ dysfunction have already been described in detail in Chapter 1:

Tenderness to palpation of TMJs and/or muscles of mastication
TMJ clicking and locking
Deviation of the mandible on opening of the mouth
Limitation of opening of the mouth.

The symptoms may be associated with:

Pain in neck and shoulders
Recurrent headaches
Ear symptoms
Vertigo
Swallowing difficulty.

Symptoms may occur in different combinations, unilaterally or bilaterally and may be present constantly or intermittently. The severity of symptoms may vary and they are typically aggravated by mandibular movement. Clicking may be present with or without pain. Diagnosis is based upon a careful history and examination which includes auscultation of TMJ's and careful interpretation of the results of palpation of TMJ's and muscles of mastication and an absence of radiographic findings on conventional views such as OPT.

PAIN/TENDERNESS

Localized muscle pain can occur in firm nodules or bands of muscles or tendons termed trigger points. One or several muscles may be affected unilaterally or bilaterally. The condition may also be more diffuse and the muscles may appear slightly swollen. There may be slight reddening of the skin over the affected area and the mandibular mobility is often limited. Prolonged habitual clenching of the teeth may lead to masseter muscle hypertrophy with or without pain.

Reflex splinting due to pain or muscle spasm may severely *limit mandibular* opening in severe cases.

Unfavourable forces on the TMJ may result in damage and inflammation of the capsule, capsular ligaments or synovial membranes of the TMJ. This will be associated with a varying degree of tenderness to palpation of the lateral or posterior aspects of the TMJ and with painful mandibular movement.

CLICKING, LOCKING AND DISC DISPLACEMENT

Clicking may occur in the absence of pain. This has been described in Chapter 1. Klineberg (1991) has reviewed possible causes of clicking and has described the features associated with each type (Table 5.1). Dysfunction of lateral pterygoid or masseter muscles may lead to uncoordinated movement of the TMJ disc resulting in joint clicking, but the most common cause is disc displacement.

DISC DISPLACEMENT

Whilst the term internal derangement might be used to describe any intra-articular pathology it is usually used to describe anterior or antero-medial TMJ disc displacement. More rarely the disc may be displaced posteriorly or anterolaterally. Anterior disc displacement may be difficult to distinguish clinically from other forms of TMJ dysfunction and confirmation may only be obtained with a reason-

Table 5.1 TMJ clicking (after Klineberg, 1991)

Dysfunction	Clinical signs
(i) Click associated with deviation in form of condyle	Opening and closing click in same position in opening and closing movement
(ii) Click associated with neuromuscular dysfunction	Opening click at a variable position in opening
(iii) Eminence click (hard)	Opening click middle to late in opening
(iv) Click (reciprocal) with anterior disc displacement	Opening click early Closing click late
(v) Click (soft) associated with hypermobility	Opening click late
(vi) Tethered disc	Opening and closing click moderate opening

able degree of certainty by arthrography or MRI. Thus, it is often included in the clinical 'umbrella' diagnosis of TMJ dysfunction. However, since treatment may differ it deserves separation for both descriptive and diagnostic purposes.

Anterior disc displacement
Anterior disc displacement (with reduction) has been described in Chapter 1 and is associated with reciprocal clicking which may be painful and can be associated with any of the other symptoms of TMJ dysfunction, especially irregularity or restriction of jaw movement. Confirmation of disc displacement can only be obtained by arthrography which is invasive, or by MRI which is expensive and not widely available. Difficulty in making a positive diagnosis leads cases of anterior disc displacement with reduction to be included in a less specific clinical diagnosis of TMJ dysfunction, but disc dislocation can be suspected on clinical grounds, i.e. by the presence of reciprocal clicking or locking.

The diagnosis of anterior disc displacement (without reduction) is derived from the history (clicking which has suddenly disappeared and been replaced by limitation of opening), clinical examination (reduced mouth opening with deviation of the mandible to the affected side during mouth opening, pain from the TMJ during active or passive mouth opening) and radiographic examination (increased space between the articular eminence and condyle in maximal mouth opening position, reduced anterior mobility of the condyle), or arthrography showing the displaced position and the changed configuration of the disc.

Posterior disc displacement
A posteriorly dislocated disc is associated with difficulties in closing the teeth together and TMJ pain on tooth clenching. This is an uncommon clinical condition.

TMJ dislocation

Condylar dislocation occurs when the head of the condyle passes over the articular eminence and is locked in this position by muscular forces which prevent the condyle returning into the articular fossa. Patients often experience an intense panic sensation when this occurs. Diagnosis of a condylar dislocation is made from the history (the mouth is suddenly locked in the wide open position) and clinical examination where the condyles can be palpated in a position anterior of the fossae. In unilateral cases there is deviation of the mandible to the contralateral side and radiographic examination shows the affected condyle anterior to the fossa. The condition commonly occurs following a wide yawn or sometimes during dental treatment. It is probably due to laxity of the attachment of the ligaments around the joint. Hyperactivity in the lateral pterygoid and disc damage may be predisposing factors.

Recurrent dislocation of the mandible may be very distressing for the patient, although patients often learn to reposition the jaw themselves.

Arthritis

Diseases of the TMJ may cause pain and functional disturbances similar to those found in TMJ dysfunction. There are three main groups of joint diseases involving the TMJ, namely degenerative joint disease (osteoarthrosis), traumatic arthritis and inflammatory joint disease (e.g. rheumatoid arthritis).

OSTEOARTHROSIS

Osteoarthrosis (OA) of the TMJ is common and can give symptoms that are difficult to distinguish from TMJ dysfunction. Since the management of the problems differ, OA will also be considered in detail.

OA can be defined as a primary non-inflammatory disease of movable joints characterized by deterioration and abrasion of the articular soft tissue surfaces and by simultaneous remodelling processes in the underlying bone. OA generally produces symptoms in single joints of the body, including the TMJ, although generalized involvement may occur. The general state of physical health is seldom affected in this disease. Painful symptoms are attributed to secondary inflammation of the synovial membrane (synovitis) and the disease is then termed osteoarthritis.

The frequency of OA in the TMJ increases with age. However, it seldom develops before the age of 40. It is more common in females. Crepitation, which may be regarded as the most reliable clinical sign of OA of the TMJ, was noted in 24% of a population in southern Sweden. This figure is in agreement with the frequency of OA found at postmortem. The frequency of radiographic signs of OA in the TMJ has been investigated in many clinical series and figures ranging from 22 to 44% have been presented. The radiographic examination does not detect incipient OA which is not yet discernible in the mineralized tissues of the joint. (On the other hand, extensive resorption of the subarticular compact bone due to remodelling may occur in spite of an intact articulating surface, which may lead to overdiagnosis.)

The aetiology of OA is not yet entirely understood. It probably embraces both local and systemic factors. Age is a predisposing factor, but there is no evidence of any functionally important age-dependent alteration in the joint tissues which indicates that ageing plays a primary aetiologic role. The most important single aetiologic factor known is mechanical overloading of the joint. Loss of molar support has also been found to be associated with TMJ crepitation and OA of the TMJ.

Other factors which also may increase the load carried by the TMJ are muscular hyperactivity (bruxism), unilateral chewing, deformity following trauma and congenital defects. The local mechanical factors are also influenced by largely unknown systemic factors. A combination of local and systemic factors seems to determine the development and progression of OA of the TMJ and other joints.

The development of OA in the articular cartilage is followed by remodelling of the fibrocartilage and the underlying bone resulting in a deviation of shape of the bony tissues. The articular eminence and the condyle are thereby flattened and the marginal peripheral area of the condyle is hypervascularized leading to bony outgrowths (osteophytes).

OA often starts in the TMJ disc. Long-standing compressive overload here results in thinning, cell necrosis, intercellular matrix degradation and eventually perforation (Fig. 5.1). There is a vascularization in the vicinity of the perforations, which has been interpreted as a sign of repair. The thinning or perforation of the disc increases the strain on the other opposing joint compo-

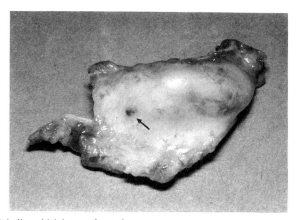

Figure 5.1 A disc which has perforated

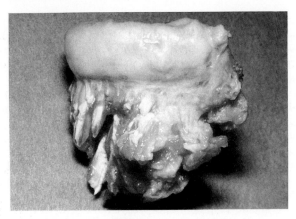

Figure 5.2 A mandibular condyle exhibiting gross osteoarthritic changes

nents, and if their adaptability is exceeded, OA develops here also (Fig. 5.2). In severe cases, the combined effect of OA and remodelling results in a severely deformed joint lacking a soft articular surface.

Symptoms of OA such as pain, stiffness and reduced mobility can often be attributed to secondary inflammation of the synovial membrane (synovitis). There are at least two different mechanisms besides trauma by which an inflammatory response can be elicited in OA of the TMJ. The degradation products from the joint surface are capable of causing a chronic synovitis, which in turn causes further destruction of the articular surface. Pyrophosphate has been found in high concentrations in the synovial fluid from joints with OA. Free crystals of pyrophosphate in the synovial fluid can elicit an acute inflammatory response.

Clinical features
The subjective symptoms and signs associated with OA of the TMJ resemble those of other forms of TMJ disorder and include pain and tenderness to palpation of the TMJ and masticatory muscles, stiffness and pain and limitation of mandibular movement. Grating noise in the TMJ on mandibular movement is an important, but relatively late, symptom. There is a generalized form of OA and so details of signs and symptoms in other joints, especially the load-bearing joints such as knees and hips, should be sought.

Radiographic findings

Radiography is a common means of diagnosing OA of the TMJ. Interpretation of the radiographs, especially the differentiation between OA and merely deviation in form of the TMJ can be difficult. The radiographic signs of reduced joint space, subcortical sclerosis and flattening of the lateral parts of the joint are characteristic of TMJ OA. The conventional radiographic methods pose problems in the interpretation of the joint space while tomography gives the most accurate information about the joint space and position of the condyle. Absence or reduction of the antero-superior joint space will indicate destruction of fibrocartilage tissue of the disc and the articular surfaces of the temporal component and condyle. If the reduced joint space is associated with joint crepitus it is very likely to be caused by fibrocartilage destruction. Marginal osseous outgrowths, known as osteophytes, are common as a result of remodelling processes and OA, as is flattening of both joint components.

TRAUMATIC ARTHRITIS

Traumatic arthritis is an inflammatory response to excessive external trauma to the joint tissues. It may be complicated by fracture of the neck of the mandible or intra-capsular fracture of the condyle. External facial trauma from blows to the mandible area transmits forces to one or both of the TMJs. Posteriorly directed forces result in a compression of the posterior, and highly innervated and vascularized attachment of the disc. The soft tissues may be torn and an intra-capsular bleeding may ensue. If the capsule and ligaments are subjected to tension, tearing of the capsule and loosening of the posterior attachment may occur. An inflammatory response develops shortly after the trauma and is characterized by increased vascular permeability leading to oedema. The joint effusion is usually clear (occasionally bloody) with a low white blood cell count.

The clinical picture is dominated by painful limitation of movement and joint swelling caused by effusion. Traumatic arthritis of the TMJ is usually unilateral. The swollen joint is very tender and the intra-articular effusion often displaces the mandible (the chin) to the contralateral side with alteration of the occlusion. The occlusion can, however, be forced back to normal by backward pressure on the chin, but it is a painful procedure. The radiographic picture of the joint is normal except for a possible widening of the joint space. Radiographic examination is important, however, to rule out the existence of mandibular fractures. The diagnosis is thus based on the clinical signs and a recent history of trauma.

RHEUMATOID ARTHRITIS

Rheumatoid arthritis (RA) is a systemic connective tissue disease of inflammatory nature. The disease may involve any joint of the body, but often starts in peripheral finger and toe joints, eventually spreading proximally to involve the large joints such as knee and shoulder joints. The extent of joint involvement and the severity of the inflammatory process can vary considerably, but often the disease has a slow, chronic course with progressive destruction of cartilage, bone and other joint tissues with weakening of the nearby muscles. This process often results in stiff and deformed joints.

Occurrence

The occurrence of TMJ symptoms caused by RA involvement depends on the severity of systemic disease, but it can be expected that every second patient with RA will experience symptoms from this joint. In Sweden, 2.5% of the population above 20 years has been reported to have RA, females being affected three times as often as males. The disease often starts in the middle-aged female. Severe forms of the disease with great functional disability occur in about 10–15% of the patients.

Clinical features

The disease usually starts in joints other than the TMJ, as do other polyarthritides. Thus patients must be asked about the existence of general joint symptoms. The subjective symptoms in RA of the TMJ include pain both at rest and on mandibular movements, stiffness in the morning, difficulty in opening the mouth and sometimes swelling. The patient can often experience a grating noise in the joint.

The most specific clinical signs of RA in the TMJ are palpatory tenderness of the joint (laterally and/or posteriorly) and crepitation (palpable or audible) from the joint. The latter is produced by destruction of the fibrocartilage and bony articular surfaces. Both these signs, however, can occur in osteoarthrosis as well as in inflammatory joint diseases. Swelling of the TMJ extending from the zygomatic arch down to the neck of the mandible can occasionally be seen. A characteristic feature of severe RA in the TMJ is a progressive development of an anterior open bite due to bilateral destruction of the mandibular condyles. The mandible is thereby rotated postero-superiorly around the molar teeth. The destruction of the joints is associated with inflammation and usually pain with functional disability. The open bite may be created in a couple of months during an acute episode of the general disease. The amount of joint destruction and the degree of anterior open bite depend on the severity of the systemic disease and varies considerably between patients. Findings of tenderness to palpation of the masticatory muscles, reduced mandibular mobility and irregular mandibular movement patterns complete the clinical picture.

There are specific blood tests for RA. The ESR (erythrocyte sedimentation rate) is raised as in other inflammatory joint diseases and may be associated with anaemia.

Radiographic findings
The most characteristic radiographic signs of RA in the TMJ are reduced joint space and severe destruction of the bone which rarely may lead to a complete loss of the condyle. The reduced joint space is caused by destruction of the articular cartilage, which results in a narrowing of the mineralized joint surfaces, and is similar to that occurring in OA. Bone sclerosis and bony outgrowths (osteophytes) may also occur, but are more characteristic of osteoarthrosis. The radiographic appearance of RA in the TMJ is therefore not specific, especially in the early phase. There is a time-lag in the development of radiographic changes as compared with the clinical symptoms.

OTHER INFLAMMATORY JOINT DISEASES

There are several other causes of inflammation in the joint including gout, psoriatic arthritis and infection.

In the acute phases of these conditions there will be signs of inflammation, the joint being painful and restricted in movement, sometimes swollen, while redness is seldom observed. These conditions are usually associated with systemic signs and symptoms.

Gout
Gout is caused by the deposition of uric acid crystals in the synovial membrane. It has a prevalence of 0.3%, males aged 30–60 years predominate and usually other joints are or have been involved before the TMJs.

Psoriatic arthritis
In recent years psoriatic arthritis has been considered to be a distinct entity. Psoriatic arthritis can be defined as an inflammatory disease of joints in a patient with psoriasis, usually with a negative serological test for rheumatoid factor. The skin lesions usually precede the arthritis. About 5–10% of the individuals with psoriasis have psoriatic arthritis and about 2% of the population in Scandinavia will suffer from psoriasis. There is probably a female

predominance of patients with psoriatic arthritis. The aetiology of psoriasis is unknown, as is the cause of joint involvement in some patients. The pathology and pathogenesis of psoriatic arthritis resembles that of rheumatoid arthritis.

Infective arthritis
Acute infective conditions of the joint are rare and can now rapidly be treated by antibiotics and damage to the joint can thereby be prevented. The increased prevalence of venereal diseases makes gonococcal arthritis a possibility that must be considered.

Ankylosis

Ankylosis produces extreme limitation of mandibular movement. Ankylosis may be due to fibrous adhesions within the joint or to bony union between joint components which results in complete immobility of the joint. It is a rare condition that is due to trauma or infection.

Neoplasia

Although tumours of the tissues of the TMJ are uncommon, case reports of benign and malignant tumours of the joint have clearly illustrated that signs and symptoms referrable to these neoplasms simulate those of TMJ dysfunction. Benign tumours are most commonly found, e.g. osteoma, chondroma and chondromatosis. Malignant tumours are very rare and are usually metastatic.

Congenital and developmental disorders

These disorders are rare.

AGENESIS

This is a developmental failure. The auditory apparatus is also usually affected.

HYPOPLASIA

Incomplete development is less severe than agenesis. It may be associated with fibrous ankylosis.

HYPERPLASIA

This overdevelopment may occur as a localized enlargement of condyle or coronoid process or as an overdevelopment of the entire mandible or side of the face. An enlarged coronoid process may cause restriction of mandibular mobility.

Differential diagnosis

- Dental pain
- Disorders of the ears, nose and sinuses
- Disorders of parotid gland
- Musculoskeletal disorders of head and neck
- Neuralgias and headaches
- Drug-induced muscle spasm
- Somatic presentations of psychiatric disease
- Angina.

Dental pain

Dental disease may sometimes be confused with TMJ dysfunction when the pain is diffuse. It is most important for the dentist to identify and eliminate possible dental causes of facial pain. Referred pain from jaw muscles (masseter and temporalis muscles) may be experienced as toothache in the molar and premolar regions of both maxilla and mandible (masseter) or maxilla only (temporalis).

Disorders of the ears, nose and sinuses

TMJ pain is often thought by the patient to be due to pathology of the ear and if there is any doubt the patient's GP or an ENT specialist should be consulted.

The most common conditions would be acute or chronic otitis media. In the former the temperature would be elevated and it generally follows an upper respiratory tract infection. The drum will be red and loss of hearing on that side noted. Chronic conditions will likewise have deafness and a discharge.

The patient's subjective symptoms of pain, tinnitus, vertigo or fullness in the ears are symptoms which may in some patients be attributed to TMJ dysfunction.

Tinnitus is a condition which is not well understood or treated, and vertigo, described by the patient as dizziness, is, in the authors' opinion, not commonly associated with TMJ dysfunction. Some doubt exists as to whether the TMJ or masticatory muscles can in fact produce such symptoms. There is some evidence that hyper-activity of the postural muscles of the head, i.e. the sternocleido-mastoid, the trapezius and deep neck muscles, is able to cause vertigo.

Disorders of the parotid gland

The parotid gland, the largest of the salivary glands is closely related to both the TMJ and the masticatory muscles (Fig. 5.3). Disorders of the parotid may produce symptoms similar to those of TMJ dysfunction.

Swelling is an important feature of salivary gland disorders but may be considered unusual in TMJ dysfunction. Pain from parotid affection often increases with increased swelling and may also be aggravated by mandibular movement, eating and swallowing. The importance of a careful examination of a swollen area is evident.

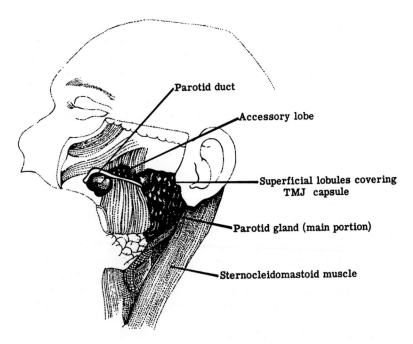

Figure 5.3 The anatomical relationship between the parotid gland, TMJ and masseter muscle

Head and neck pain from the cervical spine

It is believed that cervical disease causes headaches mediated by paraspinous cervical muscles. Noxious irritation of cervical tissues causes reflex activity through vertebral nerves.

It is not uncommon for patients complaining of TMJ pain to have associated pains in the head, neck and shoulders and this can be an important aspect of differential diagnosis in establishing whether the pain is due to the TMJ and masticatory muscles, or whether it is referred pain along the segmental nerve supply of C2 and/or C3 with symptoms of discomfort along the horizontal and ascending borders of the ramus of the mandible. It is a common distribution of TMJ pain, but the diagnosis of cervical pain can usually be established by moving the neck which results in an aggravation or relief of pain. Radiographs of the spine may be misleading since many individuals without symptoms may show evidence of degenerative changes. Referral for a medical opinion is advisable.

Neuralgias and headaches

None of the typical neuralgias (e.g. trigeminal neuralgia) are likely to be confused with TMJ or muscle pain due to their classical clinical picture. The atypical neuralgias are generally associated with vascular changes and are not well understood. They range from the classical migraine to a variety of types of headache which have been called histaminic cephalgia. Horton's or 'cluster' headache is usually found in the male (8:1) and occurs periodically with times of remission in between. The pain is severe, continual and located over the eye, and the eye is swollen and waters. It may be triggered by vasodilators, such as alcohol, and there is usually no visual changes or nausea with it to differentiate the conditions from classical migraine. They last for 30–60 minutes and recur in 24 hourly periods often waking the patient at the same time of night.

Classical migraine is more common in women than in men and there is often a family history of similar headaches. The headache is ushered in with an aura and visual disturbances. Nausea and vomiting are common at the peak of the attack which lasts for hours or days. The attack is followed by muscle tension and often pain, especially in the temporalis muscle.

It is unlikely that these conditions in their developed form would be confused with TMJ and muscle pain, but in minor forms of headache some confusion can occur.

Drug induced muscle spasm

Drugs of the phenothiazine type and the piperidine group, of which Stelazine (trifluoperazine) is the most commonly used, tend to produce stiffness and contraction of the jaw muscles, dysarthria and dysphagia. Extrapyramidal symptoms like Parkinson's disease may be seen in addition to the dyskinetic forms. Prochlorperazine has also been shown to produce dislocation of the joint.

Somatic presentations of psychiatric disorders

Somatic (physical, bodily) complaints form part of the symptom pattern in all the common primary psychiatric disorders. Anxiety states are associated with autonomic overarousal which may result in heightened muscle tension. This may produce muscular pain.

Depressive disorders may be associated with psychogenic atypical facial pain, a constant, often diffuse, poorly located facial pain that is not associated with any nerve distribution or identifiable pathology.

More severe psychiatric disorders such as obsessional neurotic or psychotic disorders result in bizarre descriptions of symptoms or single symptom delusions such as phantom bite or migratory odontalgia.

Angina

Severe ischaemic chest pain usually radiates to the left arm. Occasionally it radiates to the left mandible and rarely it is experienced in the teeth, tongue and palate. The pain is usually precipitated by exertion or by emotion such as anger or anxiety.

Further reading

Carlsson G E, Kopp S and Oberg T (1979) Arthritis and allied diseases. In: *Temporomandibular Joint. Function and Dysfunction* (Zarb G A and Carlsson G E, eds). Munksgaard, Copenhagen & Mosby, St. Louis, pp. 269–276

Cephalalgia (1988) Classification and diagnostic criteria for headache disorders, cranial neuralgias and facial pain. *Cephalalgia 8*, Supplement 7, Norwegian University Press

Christiansen E L and Thompson J R (1990) *Temporomandibular Joint Imaging.* Mosby Year Book, St. Louis

Dworkin S F and Le Resche L (1992) Research diagnostic criteria for temporomandibular disorders: Review, criteria, examinations and specifications, critique. *Journal of Craniomandibular Disorders: Facial and Oral Pain*, **6**, 301–355

Enoch M D and Jagger R G (1994) *Psychiatric Disorders in Dental Practice.* Butterworth-Heinemann, Oxford

Klineberg I (1991) *Craniomandibular Disorders and Orofacial Pain*. Wright, Oxford
Kopp S (1992) Diagnosis and nonsurgical treatment of the arthritides. Connective tissue aspects. In: *The Temporomandibular Joint. A Biological Basis for Clinical Practice* (Sarnat B G and Laskin D M, eds). W B Saunders, London, pp. 359–361
Marbach J J, Varoscak J R and Blank R T (1983) 'Phantom bite': classification and treatment. *Journal of Prosthetic Dentistry*, **49**, 556–559

6

Treatment

The history, examination and special investigations should allow the clinician to arrive at a *diagnosis*. Treatment should be based upon the diagnosis and upon an understanding of the contributing factors.

The nature and extent of the treatment will depend on the nature of the aetiological factors, the severity of the patient's symptoms and on the patient's expectations. It should be noted that it is not always possible to positively identify aetiological factors.

The aims of the management of patients with TMJ dysfunction are essentially the same as for patients with other orthopaedic or rheumatic disorders, i.e. decreased pain, decreased adverse load, restored function and restored normal daily activities (McNeil, 1993). Treatment may be palliative, preventative or curative.

Much remains to be learned about the natural course of symptoms of TMJ dysfunction, e.g. which symptoms have the most or least favourable prognosis. However, signs and symptoms may be transient or self-limiting. Irreversible, aggressive and extensive treatments such as complex occlusal reconstruction or surgical intervention should therefore always be avoided if possible and measures such as counselling and physical treatments are indicated for most patients. The great majority of patients with symptoms of temporomandibular joint dysfunction can be successfully treated in this way. The rate of recurrence of symptoms from muscular dysfunction and osteoarthrosis is not very high.

Despite good results of conservative measures, a small proportion of patients may be resistant to treatment. If treatment methods prove ineffective it is important that the original diagnosis is reassessed, since many other conditions may produce symptoms similar to TMJ dysfunction.

Those patients with TMJ dysfunction do not respond to conservative treatment measures may fall into two broad groups and should be referred to a specialist for further assessment and management:

● Those with symptoms caused by gross intra-articular pathological changes. These may be considered candidates for joint surgery.

● Patients with complex chronic 'psychogenic' facial pain. Chronic pain is a complex perceptual process where somatic and psychologic factors are intertwined. A multidisciplinary approach to the management of these patients has been recommended to address physical, psychological and psychosocial problems. Management of 'psychogenic' facial pain can include supportive psychological treatments such as antidepressant medication, behaviour therapy, hypnosis and cognitive therapies. It is therefore wise for the dental practitioner to refer patients who suffer severe chronic facial pain for specialist advice and management.

Placebo effect and the management of TMJ dysfunction

Symptoms may be relieved and/or side-effects produced by a non-active agent if a patient believes that agent to be active. This phenomenon is described as the placebo effect. The precise nature of the placebo effect is still the subject of investigation, but it is believed to be at least partly explained by release by the body of substances known as endorphins. Present evidence suggests the following:

● The placebo effect is most active when pain is severe.
● The placebo effect is reduced with continued treatment by the placebo.
● There is no proven relationship between the individual's 'suggestibility' and the placebo response.
● There is a positive relationship between anxiety and the placebo effect.
● The placebo effect may be increased by enthusiastic presentation of treatment.
● The placebo response is dependent upon the quality of the doctor–patient relationship.

Every therapeutic measure has two uncorrelated components. One is due to the placebo effect, the other to the specific action of the therapeutic technique.

The purpose of a controlled trial is to separate these components so that an estimation of the specific action of the therapeutic effect can be made.

Although the placebo effect may hinder experimental investigation, it may be used constructively as a valuable adjunct to the chosen therapeutic technique.

Treatment methods

The following types of treatments are available for symptoms of TMJ dysfunction:

● Physical
● Occlusal
● Pharmacological
● Surgical.

Physical treatments

COUNSELLING, ADVICE AND REASSURANCE

A thorough examination, including radiography, usually rules out serious disease as a cause of symptoms and the patient should be immediately reassured that the prognosis of treatment of this condition is good. Advice on how to avoid undue forces on the muscles and joints is often the most important feature of the management. Rest and relaxation are important in trying to reduce the pain and it is important that the patient prevents undue force being placed on the TMJs and muscles of mastication by avoiding damaging habits such as nail biting and tooth clenching and also avoiding chewing tough foods, yawning widely and enthusiastic incising of food.

Emotional tension and anxiety are often present in patients with pain and dysfunction. Patients sometimes fear that the symptoms which they suffer are caused by cancer or other serious diseases. Symptoms can often be considerably relieved by informing the patient of the benign character of the condition. Psychogenic magnification or intensification is a concept which describes the observed phenomenon that all pains become strong when they are on a patient's mind. The 'pain-spasm cycle' is an extension of this concept. Muscle tension produces pain which causes worry concerning the pain which causes more muscle tension, etc. Reassurance can 'break the cycle' and help resolve symptoms.

If stress is believed to be an important factor referral for stress management instruction or counselling in relaxation techniques may sometimes be a help. Environmental changes, i.e. changes in the family situation, a less stressful job etc., are often impractical, but it is nevertheless very important to take time to listen to the patient's problems.

PHYSICAL EXERCISES

Physical exercises may be used as an adjunctive therapy to relax hyperactive masticatory muscles. The aim of physical exercises is to achieve increased strength and better coordination of the muscles. The mobility of the mandible is often reduced in patients with TMJ dysfunction. Physical exercises may help to restore normal movement capacity after the healing of a mandibular fracture. There is no absolute contra-indication to physical exercises other than unhealed fractures, acute arthritis and acute infections in the facial region. However, pain provoked during or after the exercises means that exercises should be discontinued.

The mandibular movements in the exercises can be performed either freely or against resistance provided by the hands. The latter is effective in increasing the muscular strength and in relaxing the antagonistic muscles, but may provoke pain in an early phase of treatment. All three principle movements are exercised, i.e. mouth opening/closing, protrusion and lateral movement. An exercise programme should start with small, relaxed warming up movements and then be followed by maximum movements. In the next phase, resistance is applied against the movement by one or both hands (Fig. 6.1). The reciprocal inhibitory mechanism of the neuro-

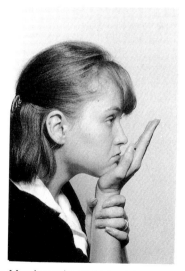

Figure 6.1 Jaw exercise. Mouth opening against resistance

muscular system results in a relaxation of the antagonist, which is supposed to be proportional to the force of the contraction of the agonist. The relaxing effect of this mechanism might then be enforced by strong resistance to the movements. Passive stretching of the closing muscles may be performed after maximum active mouth opening to increase the opening capacity and to stimulate the closing muscles to forceful contraction.

Each patient should be given an individual training programme and instructions, as well as a simple explanation of why the physical exercises should be used (see Appendix 4). The exercises should be performed preferably twice a day, in quiet surroundings. It is also recommended that tender muscles and trigger points be gently massaged.

HEAT AND COLD

Heat can be given superficially in the form of infrared waves (10–20 minutes) and hot compresses (10–20 minutes). Ethyl chloride spray can be used to chill the skin surface over the masticatory muscles. The affected muscles may be gently stretched by active movement by the patient following application. This is termed the spray-stretch technique (Fig. 6.2). It is important that the eyes, ears and nasal mucosa are protected during the application and that the skin does not become 'frosted' by excessive application. Both heat and cold applied on the skin can be used to block pain in underlying masticatory muscles and TMJ for about 20 minutes, sometimes long enough to relax the muscles. During this period, careful muscle stretch exercises should be tried in order to restore the function of the tense muscles. The analgesic effect of these two forms of treatment is probably explained by the 'gate control theory' of pain. Neither heat nor cold has a lasting effect, unless the pain–tension circle is broken, but can be of help to enable physical exercises to begin and be more effective. Heat is contra-indicated in cases of acute inflammation of the TMJ (e.g. traumatic arthritis) and of acute infection in surrounding tissues.

SHORTWAVE DIATHERMY, ULTRASOUND

The frequency of the shortwaves used for therapeutic purposes is about 27 MHz. The treatment should last for about 10–15 minutes. The analgesic effect of shortwave diathermy is supposed to be caused partly by mechanical vibration and partly by deeply penetrating thermal energy. The increase of temperature in the deep tissues may become considerable (42–45°C) and result in an important

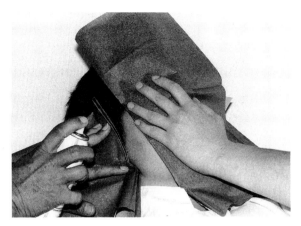

Figure 6.2 The use of an ethyl chloride spray to chill the surface of the skin over the right masseter muscle

increase of the elasticity and plasticity of the tissue collagen. This mechanism makes shortwave diathermy and ultrasonics very suitable as introductory treatments before physical exercises. They are of special importance in the treatment of spastic muscles. An increased temperature and accordingly increased blood flow can therefore be achieved also in the deeper muscles by shortwave diathermy (e.g. the lateral pterygoid). Shortwave diathermy is indicated in patients with pain in the masticatory muscles or TMJ, where temporary analgesia and muscle relaxation is needed. This treatment should, however, be followed by other more specific forms of treatment. Shortwave diathermy should not be used in the proximity of the eyes or on the TMJ during growth. Metal objects, like necklaces, earrings, should be removed from the area to be treated. Patients with pacemakers should not be treated with shortwave diathermy. Personnel should be at a distance of at least 1 metre from the apparatus and its cables. It is of help for some patients with osteoarthritis.

BIOFEEDBACK

Biofeedback mechanisms can be used as a means of relaxation training. EMG feedback has been found to be useful in reducing hyperactivity of masticatory muscles in individuals who are prone to clench their teeth during the daytime, but has been found to be less valuable in patients with nocturnal bruxism. EMG-biofeedback equipment is commercially available and includes a pair of surface electrodes made of silicone rubber, a millivoltmeter with amplifier and a visual and/or auditory display (Fig. 6.3). The concept of bio-feedback is to allow the patient to observe a physiologic response in a visual or auditory display. In training of muscle relaxation, the electric potential of the masseter muscle for instance can be recorded and displayed on a digital voltmeter so that the patient can observe the amount of muscle tension. Thus, as the masticatory muscles are tensed, a numerical increase will be observed on the millivoltmeter. During relaxation of the muscles, the figure decreases. The EMG-feedback training aims at teaching the patient to become aware of tension in the masticatory muscles and then to learn how to relax them. Successful relaxation will result in a decrease of muscle pain after a period of training.

TRANSCUTANEOUS ELECTRIC NERVE STIMULATION (TENS)

TENS can be used to achieve temporary relief of chronic localized joint and muscle pain. TENS is not useful when the pain is diffusely spread to several muscle groups or is of psychogenic origin. The duration of the analgesia is short (about 2–6 hours) unless a

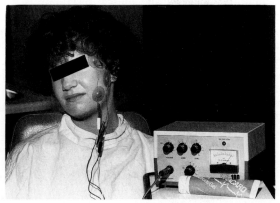

Figure 6.3 The use of an EMG (electromyographic) biofeedback equipment. The degree of muscle tension (contraction) is shown on the display in the front of the apparatus

pain–muscle tension circle is broken. The TENS has an effect similar to acupuncture, which can be at least partly explained by the 'gate control theory' of pain. The electric current stimulates a variety of receptors with low thresholds in the skin, joint and muscles (e.g. touch, temperature, pressure), which causes a massive transmission of nerve impulses via afferent large-diameter fibres, which blocks the input from the same segment of pain impulses via smaller diameter fibres. The skin overlying the painful muscles or joints is stimulated by an electric current of either high frequency (80–100 Hz) or low frequency (1–2 Hz). The current is conducted to the skin by two silicone rubber electrodes (Fig. 6.4), which are positioned on each side of the painful area. Conduction is facilitated by electrode gel. The intensity of the current (0–76 mA) is adjusted by the patient to a level just tolerated. When this level is reached, small muscle twitches may be noticed, especially with the low frequency stimulation. The stimulation is given for 20–30 minutes and analgesia is often reached after 10–20 minutes. Side-effects

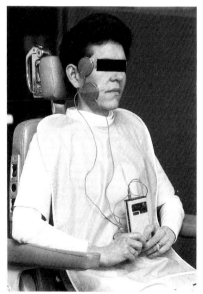

Figure 6.4 The use of transcutaneous electric nerve stimulation (TENS) equipment. The electrodes are fitted to relieve chronic pain in the right TMJ area

are rare, but temporarily increased pain and headache have been reported, as well as skin irritation if stimulation is prolonged. TENS is contra-indicated in patients with a cardiac pacemaker. This technique is usually a last resort, when the pain is chronic and is resistant to all other forms of treatment.

Occlusal treatment

OCCLUSAL SPLINTS (BITE RAISING APPLIANCES)

Symptoms in the masticatory muscles and temporomandibular joints can often be relieved by the use of an acrylic splint. The splint covers the occlusal surfaces of the teeth in the maxilla or mandible. This form of occlusal treatment has the advantage of being reversible. The mechanism whereby occlusal splints work is uncertain but several possibilities have been suggested:

● A splint encourages occlusal disengagement and reduces habitual clenching or bruxism either voluntarily or reflexly.
● Occlusal interferences are eliminated.
● Increase in occlusal vertical dimension reduces force of muscle contraction.
● The relationship of the mandibular condyle, articular disc and articular fossa is altered.

There are two main types of acrylic splints, namely those covering the whole dental arch in either jaw—stabilizing splints, and those covering the upper anterior teeth—relaxing splints.

The stabilizing splint (Fig. 6.5) is retained by extension of the acrylic beyond the survey line of the teeth and is retained like a press-stud. This type of splint can be used in either of the jaws, although the upper jaw may be preferred since it causes less encroachment on the space of the tongue. As a rule, however, the stabilizing splint is placed in the jaw with the most extensive loss of teeth. In patients with loss of posterior teeth in one of the jaws the splint can be extended to achieve occlusal contacts with the opposing jaw. In patients with a large overjet the upper jaw is preferred. Fabrication of the splint is described in Appendix 2. The splint is adjusted to give a maximum number of contacts with the opposing jaw in CR. The patient can detect whether there is even bilateral contact when the teeth are tapped gently in CR. Excursive movements should be smooth and unrestricted. On the working side there should be either cuspid protection or group contact involving the premolars and the incisors. There should be no non-working side interferences. The splint can be adjusted by self-polymerizing

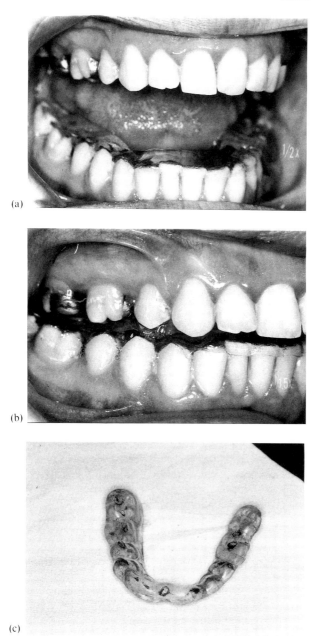

(a)

(b)

(c)

Figure 6.5 An acrylic occlusal splint. (a) Heat cured, (b) heat cured in occlusion, (c) thermoformed

acrylic resin. The splint should be as thin as possible to be comfortable, but not less than 1 mm in the posterior region due to the risk of fracture. The thickness in the anterior region will then be about 3–4 mm. A small perforation of the splint does not usually impair its function.

The stabilizing splint can be used in most patients with muscular hyperactivity and is indicated as a preventive measure in patients with advanced dental wear. There is no absolute contra-indication to this splint in adults, but it should be used with caution in children. The splint is generally recommended for use during sleep, but the time can be extended depending on the individual patient. A positive treatment effect usually appears in a week or fortnight. The splint should, however, be tried for at least a month without success before it is regarded as a treatment failure.

The occlusal splint should be checked periodically to ensure that it is not damaging the tissue of the mouth. As TMJ dysfunction resolves, jaw relationship may alter and the appliance may need further occlusal modification. Patient instructions on the use of the occlusal splint are given in Appendix 3.

The relaxing splint is a suggested alternative and is much easier to adjust, since only the anterior teeth are in occlusion with the splint. This kind of splint is not widely used and should not be used for young patients. There is a risk of anterior open bite being produced if this splint is used regularly. The stabilizing splint can easily be transformed into a relaxation splint by application of acrylic in the frontal area to disocclude the posterior teeth.

The repositioning splint is designed to provide occlusal contact with the mandible opened and protruded sufficiently so that the head of the condyle is positioned into the central cavity of the disc that is anteriorly displaced. The disc is then said to be recaptured. However, on removal of the splint the disc becomes displaced again. Its use in the treatment of anterior disc displacement reduction is described later in this chapter.

Permanent occlusal splints can be cast in cobalt-chromium and provided with an occlusal layer in acrylic (Fig. 6.6). This kind of splint is used mainly in patients with malocclusions (e.g. lateral open bite) caused by growth disturbance, arthritis, tooth loss or both. The supporting teeth are not ground and the treatment is thus reversible.

Occlusal splints are possible factors in encouraging the build up and retention of plaque resulting in caries and periodontal problems and thus should be kept scrupulously clean.

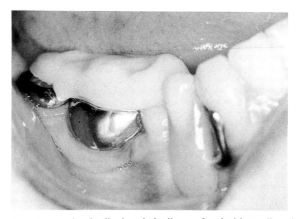

Figure 6.6 A long-term occlusal splint in cobalt alloy surfaced with acrylic resin

OCCLUSAL ADJUSTMENT

If splint treatment is successful, permanent occlusal correction may be considered. The dentist who practices irreversible correction should have a sound knowledge of the principles of occlusion and should have had instruction in the principles of occusal correction.

The objective of occlusal adjustment is to create a stable CO, with bilaterally distributed contacts between the majority of antagonizing teeth (without premature contacts in CR causing lateral or anterior displacement of the mandible) and undisturbed lateral and protrusive contact movements. Occlusal adjustment influences the pattern and degree of the sensory input from the periodontal receptors, which is the neurophysiological basis for its effect in the treatment of mandibular pain and dysfunction.

Occlusal adjustment is indicated when a causal relationship can be demonstrated between occlusal disturbances and TMJ dysfunction, or when the occlusal function *per se* is impaired and needs correction. In cases where the outcome of the adjustment is uncertain (which may be the case when a large amount of tooth structure is to be removed), mounting and analysing of models in an articulator is advisable.

Occlusal adjustment is performed using a diamond stone mounted in a dental handpiece (Fig. 6.7) with water irrigation. Indicators of thin foil, silk marking, typewriter ribbon or wax should be used to mark the exact location where the grinding should be performed. Thick articulating paper should be avoided.

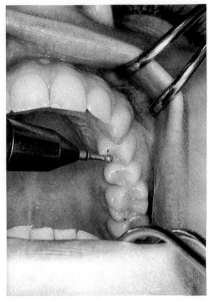

Figure 6.7 The use of diamond stones to grind marked spots on the teeth

The interferences between RCP and CO are removed by grinding according to the MUDL rule (i.e. grinding on *m*esial-*u*pper and *d*istal-*l*ower cusp facets) and the adjustment is evenly distributed between the upper and lower teeth. The adjustment is continued until the lateral displacement of the mandible is none or minimal and the occlusion in RCP is bilateral and stable. A total coincidence between CR and CO is not essential. Most often only small amounts of tooth substance need to be removed and the vertical dimension is seldom disturbed. Large sagittal distances between RCP and CO (>2 mm) are impossible to normalize entirely without extensive adjustment. In this case a reduction of the distance CR–CO and stabilization of the occlusion is preferable. A new CO is thereby created which is often perceived as an improvement in comfort by the patient.

Interferences on the non-working side during lateral excursions are removed entirely if possible, otherwise reduced as much as possible. The interference is usually localized to the palatal cusp in the upper jaw and the buccal cusp in the lower, which are both supporting cusps. The adjustment should therefore be performed on either upper or lower teeth in a way that the CO contacts remain in order to prevent elongation of the teeth involved, which can result in new interferences. The CR and CO contacts should thus be marked before adjustment. Most of the adjustment is preferably made on the palatal cusp, which is the largest. The adjustment should be continued, if possible, until contacts are achieved on the working side. If this is not possible, a reduction of the interface and thus the discrepancy on the working side is often sufficient to relieve symptoms in the masticatory muscles and TMJs.

Interfering tooth contacts during protrusive excursions which prevent incisal contact and an edge-to-edge position during incision should also be removed. Interfering cusps are adjusted in both jaws, but care should be taken not to eliminate tooth contacts in CO and CR.

Interferences which restrict or disturb protrusive or lateral excursions in the incisal region or on the working side should also be eliminated within a function range of 2 mm of CO.

Before polishing, a check is made of the tooth contacts in CO and the patient is asked whether the occlusal contacts are evenly and comfortably distributed between the right and left sides. A follow-up should be performed within two weeks and small additional adjustments may then be necessary. Malocclusions may be corrected by orthodontic treatment when indicated.

PROSTHETIC TREATMENT

Prosthetic treatment of TMJ dysfunction may follow treatment with a diagnostic splint. The aim is both to create a bilaterally stable occlusion with a sufficient number of occlusal contacts approximately 1 mm anterior to RCP on a sagittal path and to improve function. Pain and dysfunction in the TMJ and masticatory muscles may appear as a result of ill-fitting complete dentures. If there are acute symptoms the dentures may be temporarily relined and occlusal deficiencies corrected with acrylic resin on the occlusal surfaces of the lower dentures. The occlusal surfaces of the upper denture are covered with vaseline to prevent sticking to the self-polymerizing resin. The mandible with the lower denture *in situ* is carefully guided into a hinge axis closure to gently contact the upper denture before the acrylic is completely set. The lower denture is then removed and adjusted to an acceptable occlusion. This procedure is often sufficient to relieve the symptoms caused by deficient complete denture occlusion. New dentures can then be provided. In a similar manner, partial dentures can be temporarily adjusted to provide a functional occlusion.

Pharmacologic treatment

Pharmacologic treatment of symptoms of TMJ dysfunction should be used as an adjunct to other methods of management.

ANTI-INFLAMMATORY DRUGS

Acute pain may be relieved by the use of a variety of drugs. Aspirin possesses both analgesic and anti-inflammatory properties. The non-steroidal anti-inflammatory drugs (NSAID) such as ibuprofen, piroxicam, naproxen and mefenamic acid are also useful in obtaining pain relief.

ANTI-ANXIETY DRUGS AND RELAXING AGENTS

Muscular hyperactivity may be caused by emotional tension and anxiety. Anti-anxiety drugs, together with other drugs with primarily muscle relaxing properties may therefore be useful. This kind of treatment for facial pain should be short term only. Another disadvantage of treatment with tranquillizers and muscle-relaxing agents is side-effects like fatigue, drowsiness etc., which make car driving dangerous and working difficult. Use of these drugs must not be a substitute for other measures.

ANTI-DEPRESSANTS

Tricyclic anti-depressants such as dothiepin (Prothiaden) 10–30 mg at night may be effective in some cases of TMJ dysfunction that are resistant to other conservative measures. If tricyclic anti-depressants are not effective the use of monoamine oxidase inhibitors may be considered. Neither of these classes of drugs can be prescribed by a dentist by NHS prescription. The dentist may wish to ask the patient's GP to provide this treatment.

Many drugs have more than one mode of action and it is not necessarily the case that these drugs work by an anti-depressant effect. They are also of use in the treatment of atypical facial pain and oral dysaesthesias such as idiopathic burning mouth.

INTRA-MUSCULAR INJECTION

Intra-muscular injection of a local anaesthetic such as lignocaine or the longer acting bupivicaine (Marcain) may be performed in some of the masticatory muscles to obtain analgesia which may result in muscle relaxation and thereby more permanent pain relief. Injections are indicated in cases of severe localized muscle pain and tenderness and should be followed by gentle physical exercises to restore the function of the muscle. Injections can be performed without difficulty into the temporalis and masseter muscles, especially the superficial portion of the masseter and the insertion of the temporalis muscle on the coronoid process. The intraoral route is preferred and the technique is similar to that used for mandibular blocks. The most tender portion of the muscle is determined by palpation and the injection is made in that portion. The patient can often be helpful and tell if the needle reaches the most tender area. From a diagnostic point of view, intra-muscular injection of a local anaesthetic is a valuable tool to determine whether the muscle is the origin of pain. The use of a vasoconstrictor is not advocated as it may impair the blood circulation of the muscle.

INTRA-ARTICULAR INJECTIONS

The use of intra-articular injections of corticosteroids has been recommended on a limited basis in cases of severe joint pain when conservative measures have been unsuccessful. This may avoid the need for surgical intervention. Usually not more than three injections are recommended in one year since it is believed that more than this may promote degenerative changes of the articular cartilage.

Surgical treatment

Surgical procedures on the TMJ are indicated for few patients with TMJ pain and dysfunction. The following criteria are adapted from recommendations of the American Academy of Oral and Maxillo-facial Surgeons (1984) as being possible indications for surgery:

1. Documented TMJ disc displacement or other structural joint disorder with appropriate imaging.
2. Positive evidence to suggest that the symptoms and objective findings are a result of disc displacement or other structural disorders.
3. Pain or dysfunction of such magnitude as to constitute a disability to the patient.
4. Prior unsuccessful non-surgical treatment that includes occlusal splint therapy, physical therapy and behaviour therapy.
5. Prior management of bruxism, oral parafunctional habits, other medical or dental conditions, and other contributing factors that will affect outcome of surgery.

6. Patient consent after a discussion of potential complications, goals to achieve, success rate, timing, postoperative management, and alternative approaches including no treatment.

Surgery is contra-indicated when facial pain is diffuse or is mainly localized to an area other than the TMJ. It is also contra-indicated when psychiatric factors are suspected as playing a significant aetiological role.

There are four major operative procedures used on the TMJ, namely menisectomy, procedures for disc repositioning, condylectomy and condylotomy. *Menisectomy* in osteoarthrosis involves the removal of damaged/inflamed disc and capsular tissues, which are the source of pain. Removal of the perforated TMJ disc does not usually result in any disturbance of the occlusion, but extensive remodelling of the mineralized parts of the joint can occur later. There is a potential risk of future osteoarthrotic damage of the joint cartilage as a result of the removal of a normal disc. However most discs removed from joints with osteoarthrosis or rheumatoid arthritis are severely damaged and cannot therefore be of any significant functional value.

Disc repositioning operations have been developed for those patients with persistent clicking or when the disc has locked anteriorly or posteriorly. The position of the disc is ascertained by single or double contrast arthrography and, if conservative treatment fails and the symptoms are still severe, surgical treatment can be considered. An anteriorly dislocated disc may be repositioned and resutured to its posterior attachment and deviations in shape of the articular eminence and mandibular condyle can be surgically recontoured. The TMJ disc should normally be biconcave in the sagittal plane, but is frequently changed to a round or biconvex form as a sequelae of the displacement (soft-tissue remodelling). A displaced disc which is biconcave can be repositioned surgically to its normal position, while the displaced disc of biconvex shape must be removed to relieve the locking. Disc repositioning is indicated for relatively few patients.

Condylectomy involves the removal of the mandibular condyle or part of it (high condylectomy) and is performed when severe destruction and deviation in shape of the joint are present, as in degenerative or inflammatory joint disease, and in cases of ankylosis. Total condylectomy affects the occlusion with a tendency to create an open bite on the contralateral side.

Condylotomy is a closed surgical procedure that might be indicated in osteoarthrosis and is performed in order to change the loading condition in the joint. The change in loading is created by an artificial fracture of the condylar neck. Occlusal adjustment is usually necessary on the operated side.

When surgery is indicated the long-term success rate can be expected to be high, although patients may have some persistent clinical symptoms postoperatively that need further conservative treatment. Facial nerve damage is a potentially serious complication.

Management of common disorders

It is important that the management of the patient with symptoms of TMJ dysfunction is tailored to the patient's needs, expectations and severity and duration of the symptoms. It must be emphasized again that the majority of TMJ symptoms are mild and transient. Simple reassurance and a careful explanation to the patient of the nature of the condition will often be sufficient.

If symptoms fail to respond to the selected conservative measures and pain persists or if joint sounds remain very troublesome, referral for specialist care is recommended. Early referral of complex chronic TMJ facial pain patients is also recommended.

Common disorders:

● Acute traumatic damage
● Clicking
● TMJ pain dysfunction
● Anterior disc displacement
    with reduction (reciprocal click)
    without reduction (closed lock)
● Dislocations
● Arthritis.

Acute traumatic damage

Treatment of acute joint damage includes avoidance of mandibular movement, soft diet and use of analgesic and anti-inflammatory drugs. Physical exercises may be indicated after the acute stage to restore mandibular mobility and muscle power. Acute symptoms often subside spontaneously within a week and recovery is often complete within a month.

Clicking

Treatment of clicking is often disappointing. It is unwise to draw a patient's attention to otherwise asymptomless joint sounds.

Four basic types of treatment have been suggested:

- Reassurance regarding harmlessness
- Exercises
- Splints
- Surgery.

REASSURANCE

Because clicks are often intermittent and may resolve spontaneously it may be sufficient to explain the probable mechanism and to reassure the patient about its benign nature. Because a click associated with hypermobility occurs only with wide mouth opening it is sufficient to recommend that this is avoided.

EXERCISES

Jaw exercises may be useful for clicking which is due to muscle dysfunction. The patient must be advised to stop the exercises if they provoke pain (Appendix 4).

SPLINTS

Occlusal splint—An interocclusal splint may also be useful in treating a click that is due to muscle dysfunction, for example in association with habitual clenching. The use of the repositioning splint for the anteriorly displaced disc is described below.

SURGERY

Surgical treatment for a very loud click associated with an anterior disc displacement with reduction or a tethered disc may occasionally be considered necessary.

TMJ pain dysfunction

The signs and symptoms of TMJ dysfunction, like many musculo-skeletal conditions, may be transient and self-limiting. Conservative measures, avoiding aggressive intervention, should be used for the initial management of most patients. Treatment plans should be formulated taking into account predisposing, initiating and perpetuating factors as well as the wishes and expectations of the patient. All patients should be fully informed of the nature of the condition in order to alleviate anxiety. Combinations of the physical, pharmacological and occlusal treatments described above may be recommended depending on the severity of the symptoms.

A full-coverage occlusal splint may be provided if there is no early improvement in symptoms. In addition, if symptoms are severe, physical treatments and analgesics or anxiolytic drugs may be used. If these treatments are successful, permanent occlusal correction, including the removal of any occlusal interferences, may be considered, especially if symptoms recur when occlusal splint treatment is stopped.

Anterior disc displacement (ADD)

The treatment outcome for patients with disc displacement with reduction is the same as for other TMJ dysfunction patients. Painless and satisfactory function may be possible although the disc remains displaced. Clicking may be a persistent problem.

ANTERIOR DISC DISPLACEMENT WITH REDUCTION (RECIPROCAL CLICK)

Patients experiencing pain and dysfunction as a result of anterior disc displacement with reduction may be treated similarly to those with TMJ pain dysfunction as described above.

An alternative, more controversial method has been recommended by some clinicians in the USA and Scandinavia. This involves the use of a repositioning splint.

The head of the condyle may be repositioned to the central cavity of the displaced disc and therefore to a normal relationship with the disc by use of such an appliance. This means a new mandibular position with an increased vertical dimension and more protrusive. It is essential that the appliance should be worn at all times including eating. It has been shown however that the use of the appliance will not result in permanent correction of the condyle disc relationship. It has been recommended therefore that if a repositioning device has been successful then the occlusion should be permanently altered by crown and bridge, prosthetic or orthodontic treatment. This is clearly an enormous economic proposition. It should also be noted that orthodontic treatment may relapse and this form of treatment has not achieved widespread acceptance. Surgical recapture of the disc may be indicated for a few patients with severe symptoms that prove resistant to conservative measures, but relapse has been frequent.

ANTERIOR DISC DISPLACEMENT WITHOUT REDUCTION (CLOSED LOCK)

Patients may present with symptoms typical of anterior disc displacement without reduction (closed lock), described in Chapter 1. Manipulative replacement of the displaced disc may be achieved for some patients. This is done by gripping the mandible with thumbs on lower molars and distracting the condyle by pulling downward and forward. It has been recommended that if manipulation is successful, an occlusal splint should be fitted as soon as possible in order to prevent the disc displacing once again.

If the displaced disc cannot be permanently repositioned, conservative management by means of rest and occlusal splints may achieve sufficient comfort for the patient, otherwise surgical intervention must be considered as described in this chapter.

Dislocation

A dislocation of the mandible (when the mandibular condyle is unable to return to the temporal fossa) is corrected by manipulation alone if it has occurred recently. If a week or more has elapsed since the occurrence, periarticular injections of local anaesthetic are often needed to reduce the pain and muscle spasm around the joint. If these measures fail, the repositioning must be performed with sedation or general anaesthesia. Jaw exercises may be of help to prevent recurrent dislocation.

Recurrent dislocation of the mandible is treated by conservative methods first, i.e. physical (jaw) exercises and avoidance of excessive opening. A mouth prop may be used during dental procedures to help to prevent overopening of the mouth and help to support the mandible. Surgical treatment is indicated in a few cases when conservative measures fail and frequent dislocations occur. The use of sclerosing agents is not advocated.

Arthritis

OSTEOARTHRITIS (OA)

Functional overloading during mastication or bruxism plays a role in the aetiology of OA in the TMJ. Any treatment capable of reducing the strain on the TMJ is indicated. This means that habitual grinding/clenching of the teeth should be minimized. The most effective and simplest treatment is the conventional occlusal splint made of acrylic resin. The role played by occlusal interferences in bruxism and TMJ OA is uncertain, but gross interferences should be eliminated. Loss of molar support is probably a common cause of TMJ overloading. Replacement of lost molar support is therefore an objective in patients with OA of the TMJ, either by fixed bridges or partial dentures. The principles of occlusal rehabilitation are the same in OA as in other forms of TMJ disorder. Physical exercise is a good supplementary form of treatment of OA of the TMJ. It prevents muscular atrophy, diminishes the risk of capsular contraction and restores the mandibular mobility. Rest, heat and soft food may help ease pain and supplement other treatments. Heat treatment by infrared waves and shortwave diathermy have a beneficial effect in some patients, but the effect is not predictable. In OA cases with moderate to severe pain it is often useful to prescribe an analgesic drug such as salicyclic acid initially to make the patients more comfortable until further treatment can be given. Pain in joints with OA caused by an inflammatory component necessitates the use of a drug with both analgesic and anti-inflammatory properties, e.g. naproxen 250–500 mg bd, mefenamic acid 500 mg tds.

Intra-articular injection of corticosteroid is indicated in patients with severe pain caused by secondary synovitis. It can often be used successfully as treatment of patients with persistent TMJ pain due to OA in whom conventional therapy has failed. Surgical treatment is indicated in patients with long-standing severe local pain in the TMJ with both clinical (palpatory tenderness or crepitation) and radiographic evidence of TMJ OA and who do not respond to other treatment.

In the majority of patients relief can be produced by conservative measures, including occlusal splints, occlusal adjustment, physical exercises, infrared and shortwave diathermy.

RHEUMATOID ARTHRITIS (RA)

The treatment aims are to alleviate pain, reduce inflammation, restore function and, if possible, to prevent further destruction of the joints. The pain is associated with inflammation and anti-inflammatory analgesics should therefore be prescribed, if necessary. If the pain and suffering is acute an intra-articular injection of a corticosteroid often gives efficient relief, although in most cases only temporary. The prevention of further destruction is difficult, but synovectomy (surgical removal of the inflamed synovial membrane) may be performed in the TMJ as in other joints of the body. It may also improve function by removal of fibrous adherences between the joint components. The number of patients needing surgery is low, however, and most patients can be treated by conservative means. When the pain has subsided, physical exercises are indicated to improve joint–muscle function and strength. The exercises should be started gradually. The effect of heat is unpredictable, but could sometimes be used as a supplementary measure before physical exercises. Transcutaneous electric nerve stimulation (TENS) has been used for rheumatoid joint pain with good results.

The role played by the occlusion is controversial, but the general opinion is that the occlusion should be stable and free from interferences to exclude the possibility of aggravating the condition in the joint. The bone destruction in the joint occurs mainly in the functional parts of the joint, i.e. the anterior-superior part of the condyle and the infero-posterior part of the eminence. Anterior open bite caused by RA is an occlusal problem, which should be solved according to the common principles of selective grinding and prosthetic rehabilitation. However, the patient's physician should be consulted to obtain information about the disease activity before any irreversible prosthetic treatment begins. It is not advisable to make any permanent prosthetic treatment on a patient with uncontrolled RA. The treatment of patients with RA involving the TMJ is the task of both dental surgeon (local treatment) and physician (systemic treatment).

CRYSTAL DEPOSITION DISEASES

Crystal deposition diseases are inflammatory in nature and are caused by deposition of crystals in the synovial membrane. The crystals are also released into the joint cavity where they elicit an acute inflammatory reaction in the synovial membrane.

The general treatment includes anti-inflammatory drugs like phenylbutazone and indomethacin. Long-term treatment of colchicine is given to prevent the acute attacks. Drugs that lower the serum uric acid titre are also available (e.g. probenecid). The treatment of gout in the TMJ is aimed at reducing the acute local inflammatory activity either by systemic administration of anti-inflammatory drugs or by intra-articular injection of glucocorticosteroid. Mandibular rest, e.g. soft food, should be recommended during the acute attacks. The occlusion is of secondary importance with respect to the TMJ symptoms, but it should be stable and free from interferences to exclude the risk of overloading the joint.

PSORIATIC ARTHRITIS

The general treatment of psoriatic arthritis is similar to gout, i.e. anti-inflammatory medication. Acute attacks in the TMJ may also be treated by intra-articular injection of glucocorticosteroid. The occlusion should be stabilized if necessary and interferences removed in order to avoid overloading the diseased tissues.

Further reading

American Association of Oral and Maxillofacial Surgeons (1984) Position paper on TMJ Surgery. Ad hoc Committee, Chicago

Clark G T, Mohl N D and Riggs R R (1988) Occlusal adjustment therapy. In: *A Textbook of Occlusion* (N D Mohl, G A Zarb, G E Carlsson and J D Rugh, eds). Quintessence, Chicago, pp. 285–303

Holzman A D and Turk D C (1986) *Pain Management. A Handbook in Psychological Treatment Approaches*. Pergamon Press, New York

Klineberg I (1991) *Craniomandibular Disorders and Orofacial Pain*. Wright, Oxford

Kopp S (1992) Diagnosis and nonsurgical treatment of the arthritides. Connective tissue aspects. In: *The Temporomandibular Joint. A Biological Basis for Clinical Practice* (B G Sarnat and D M Laskin, eds). W B Saunders, Philadelphia, pp. 361–370

Levine J D, Gordon N C and Fields H L (1978) The mechanism of placebo analgesia. *Lancet*, **ii**, 654–657

McNeill C (1993) *Craniomandibular Disorders. Guidelines for Classification, Assessment and Management*, 2nd edn. American Academy of Orofacial Pain. Quintessence, Chicago

Mejersjö C and Carlsson G E (1985) Long term results of treatment for temporomandibular pain dysfunction. *Journal of Prosthetic Dentistry*, **49**, 809–815

Tyrer S P (1992) *Psychology, Psychiatry and Chronic Pain*. Butterworth-Heinemann, Oxford

Wise M D (1986) *Occlusion and Restorative Dentistry for the General Practitioner*, 2nd edn. British Dental Journal, London

Zarb G A and Carlsson G E (1988) The therapeutic concepts: an overview. In: *A Textbook of Occlusion* (N D Mohl, G A Zarb, G E Carlsson and J D Rugh, eds). Quintessence, Chicago, pp. 265–270

Appendix 1

International Headache Society's classification and diagnostic criteria for headache disorders, cranial neuralgias and facial pain (from *Cephalalgia,* **8** (Suppl. 7), 1988)

1. Migraine
2. Tension-type headache
3. Cluster headache and chronic paroxysmal hemicrania
4. Miscellaneous headaches, unassociated with structural lesion
5. Headache associated with head trauma
6. Headache associated with vascular disorders
7. Headache associated with non-vascular intracranial disorders
8. Headache associated with substances or their withdrawal
9. Headache associated with non-cephalic infection
10. Headache associated with metabolic disorder
11. *Headache or facial pain associated with disorder of cranium, neck, eyes, ears, nose, sinuses, teeth, mouth, or other facial or cranial structures*
12. Cranial neuralgias, nerve trunk pain, and deafferentation pain
13. Headache not classifiable

Recommended classification for category 11 modified by American Academy of Orofacial Pain*

11.1 *Cranial bones including mandible*
11.2 Neck
11.3 Eyes
11.4 Ears
11.5 Nose and sinuses
11.6 Teeth and related oral structures
11.7 *Temporomandibular joint disorders*
11.8 *Masticatory muscle disorders*

Recommended   diagnostic   classification   for   category   11.1*
(cranial bones including mandible)

11.1.1   Congenital and developmental disorders
    11.1.1.1   Agenesis
    11.1.1.2   Hypoplasia
    11.1.1.3   Condyloysis
    11.1.1.3   Hyperplasia
    11.1.1.4   Dysplasia
    11.1.2.1   Neoplasia
    11.1.2.2   Fracture

Recommended diagnostic classification for category 11.7* (temporomandibular joint disorders)
11.7.1   Deviation in form
11.7.2   Disc displacement
    11.7.2.1   Disc displacement with reduction
    11.7.2.2   Disc displacement without reduction
11.7.3   Dislocation
11.7.4   Inflammatory conditions
    11.7.4.1   Synovitis
    11.7.4.2   Capsulitis
11.7.5   Arthritides
    11.7.5.1   Osteoarthrosis
    11.7.5.2   Osteoarthritis
    11.7.5.3   Polyarthritides
11.7.6   Ankylosis
    11.7.6.1   Fibrous
    11.7.6.2   Bony

Recommended diagnostic classification for category 11.8* (masticatory muscle disorders)
11.8.1   Myofascial pain
11.8.2   Myositis
11.8.3   Spasm
11.8.4   Protective splinting
11.8.5   Contracture
11.8.6   Neoplasia

* McNeill C (ed.) (1993) *Temporomandibular Disorders. Guidelines for Classification Assessment and Management*. The American Academy of Orofacial Pain, 2nd edn. Quintessence, Chicago

Appendix 2

Constructing an occlusal splint

A splint may be made for upper or lower jaws but the principles and construction techniques are basically the same. Dental impressions of upper and lower teeth are taken in alginate or elastomer. The impressions may be accompanied by facebow and occlusal records.

The impressions are cast in 100% stone or die stone. Casts should be mounted on an average-value or semi-adjustable articulator in centric occlusion or using the occlusal records. The incisal pin is set to the desired increased occlusal vertical dimension, usually allowing approximately 1–2 mm interocclusal space in the molar region. This provides adequate thickness which will be tolerable by the patient but will allow for any further occlusal adjustment without the possibility of perforation. A wax-up of the splint is produced, building in the desired features:

1. Correct extension
2. Smooth occlusal plane
3. No interferences in centric occlusion
4. Anterior guidance
5. Canine guidance

It should be noted that an occlusal splint can also be made without the ramping that provides anterior and canine guidance and some dentists prefer this design. However, no posterior or non-working interferences should occur during mandibular excursions.

Excessive undercuts are blocked out. Baseplate wax is softened and adapted to the cast and trimmed to the required extension. For the mandibular splint this may be two-thirds of the sulcus depth lingually and overlapping buccally by approximately 2 mm, and contoured so as not to interfere with the tongue and cheeks. This should provide sufficient extension for retention. Additional retention may be gained by using stainless steel cribs or ball-ended clasps. All occlusal and incisal surfaces must be covered in order to prevent unwanted over-eruption of uncovered teeth.

The same principles apply to the maxillary splint with corresponding extension over the palate in a horseshoe shape in order to provide retention and rigidity. A pin-line post-dam is provided. The occlusal surface is contoured to a smooth occlusal plane with freedom of movement around centric occlusion and no interferences at the set vertical dimension. The anterior guidance is added in the form of a ramp/incline which provides posterior disclusion during protrusion of the mandible. Similarly, a ramp for canine guidance is added to remove non-working side interferences during lateral excursion. On completion of the wax-up the splint is invested and processed in clear heat-cured acrylic resin. It is deflasked, polished and is ready for insertion.

Alternatively, the splint may be thermoformed in a thermoplastic material. The thermoformed splint should be trimmed and replaced on the articulator for occlusal correction.

Once correctly seated, occlusal foil or articulating paper of minimal thickness is used to check occlusal contacts in centric relation, lateral excursions and in protrusion. Any interferences are removed and the occlusal surface is repolished.

Appendix 3

Patient instructions for the use of an occlusal splint

Purpose of the splint

The use of the splint is an important part of the treatment of disorders of the temporomandibular joint and chewing muscles. Its purpose is usually to give stability to the bite, reduce the load on the joint and to provide relaxation for the chewing muscles. It may also be used to prevent excessive wear of the teeth.

Use

The splint is worn for a limited period which may vary from a couple of weeks to some months, depending upon the response to the treatment. It is usually worn only at night but can sometimes be used during the day if symptoms are severe.

Possible difficulties

Several problems may arise when the splint is worn. It may feel large and clumsy and produce nausea or excessive saliva. Because of tension in the plastic some teeth may become a little tender especially in the mornings. Cheek biting may also occur. These problems usually disappear quickly with continued use of the splint. If these problems remain after a couple of days and are so bad that the splint cannot be worn, then further adjustment by the dentist is necessary. Sometimes when the splint is taken out of the mouth in the morning, the bite might not feel 'right'. This is due to the relaxation in the chewing muscles and usually indicates that slight correction of the bite is necessary for better stability.

Oral hygiene and care of the splint

Before the splint is put in the mouth, make sure that the teeth are brushed carefully. The plastic splint can also attract a layer of bacteria from the mouth and so this too should be cleaned daily—most easily with toothbrush and paste. When the splint is not being used it should be kept in water.

Appendix 4

Jaw muscle exercises

The jaw muscle exercise programme is as follows:

1. Relax and lower your shoulders.
2. Let your lower jaw relax and make an M sound. Make sure that the teeth do not contact. Relax your tongue.
3. Make small, relaxed up-and-down and side-to-side movements of the jaw without tooth contact to warm up the muscles.
4. Open and close your mouth as much as you can without pain or discomfort. Move your jaw as far as possible forward and then back. Make similar movements towards both sides and then relax.
5. Make the same movements as in exercise No. 4 but against resistance with your hand, e.g. push your fist below the jaw during opening, push your thumb against your chin during forward movement and against the right and left side of your chin during side movements. Keep your jaw at the extreme point of movement for a few seconds.
6. Open your mouth as wide as possible, then try to close while you resist this movement by pushing downward against your lower front teeth with your fingers. Hold the jaw in this position for a few seconds.
7. Open your mouth as wide as you can. Then stretch further by pushing your fingers against the front teeth of the upper and lower jaws. Relax.
8. While looking in the mirror, try to move your lower jaw straight up and down. Avoid deviations as well as movements that produce clicking or locking of the jaw.
9. End the exercise programme by resting on your back for 5 to 10 minutes.

Each exercise should be performed about 10 times and the whole training programme should be performed twice a day, unless otherwise prescribed. Movements that cause pain should be avoided. Application of heat locally over the TMJs and cheeks often makes

the exercise easier and more comfortable due to increased elasticity
of the tissues and increased local blood circulation.

Index